Pursued by a Bear

Pursued by a Bear

Or

How I Endured Years of Medical Treatment and Lived to Write About It

Paul Singer

iUniverse, Inc.
Bloomington

PURSUED BY A BEAR
Or How I Endured Years of Medical Treatment and Lived to Write About It

Copyright © 2011 by Paul Singer.

iUniverse books may be ordered through booksellers or by contacting:

iUniverse
1663 Liberty Drive
Bloomington, IN 47403
www.iuniverse.com
1-800-Authors (1-800-288-4677)

ISBN: 978-1-4620-3912-8 (sc)
ISBN: 978-1-4620-3911-1 (ebk)

Printed in the United States of America

iUniverse rev. date: 08/13/2011

Contents

In which I, a man healthy until this moment, whose background is herein described, am bestowed three medical diagnoses, two of which I know to be fatal

In which I learn more about my diagnoses, and am prescribed drugs for one and surgery is scheduled for another

In which surgery takes place and I face challenging adventures while in the hospital

In which, after my discharge from the hospital, I try a number of approaches to my medical condition and the problems that that condition causes, none of which approaches makes me feel any better

In which a miracle takes place and a new drug makes me feel better and not as though I am about to die, but not enough better to reduce my wish to try an additional drug, which no one will prescribe for me

For
Justin and Alexandra

Weep I cannot,
But my heart bleeds . . . . Farewell!
The day frowns more and more . . . .
. . . . I never saw
The heavens so dim by day. A savage clamor!
Well may I get aboard! This is the chase:
I am gone forever.   [*Exit, **pursued by a bear***

William Shakespeare.   A Winter's Tale   III, 3

Acknowledgements

I am very grateful to all my friends and family who read the manuscript at various stages of its creation and who gave thoughtful suggestions and corrected errors. I want especially to thank Diana, my beautiful and glamorous wife, for her encouragement and support during both the writing and the events I write about.

Introduction

During a twelve year period, I was inundated with frightening medical diagnoses and sometimes harsh treatments. It seemed like: name a cancer, I got it. It felt as though I couldn't turn around without some new medical problem stopping me in my tracks. "Enough already" was my mantra. It seemed that my life revolved around medical appointments and getting prescriptions filled. A handful of pills every morning and disrobing before strangers became my way of life. I was very concerned and even angry about the treatment I was getting and about whether or not the medical personnel I dealt with functioned at a level I defined as good. I wanted not only the latest high-level medical care; I wanted also to be treated nicely, thoughtfully, humanely, and with honesty, and I was sadly surprised by and came to be preoccupied with how frequently the niceties that you expect in ordinary, every-day human contacts were missing.

I did not enjoy these preoccupations of mine, these constant irritations, but since I was so often feeling so lousy and since my time was so occupied with seeing doctors and getting medical procedures done and since these preoccupations acted fortuitously sometimes to block my obsessing about what could have been very disturbing thoughts in relation to my mortality, they were hard to resist. God knows, it felt better to rage at slights, than to stay awake nights worrying about my impending death.

Whatever psychological needs I filled in the formation and preservation of these observations and obsessions, however, the slights, and they were often considerably more than slight, were real indeed and cannot be discounted. As a matter of fact, they seem, in retrospect, to typify the manner in which medical care tends to be delivered here.

In addition, the medical system's peculiarities, its proclivity to surprise around every corner with foolishness and with rigid ritual, the frequent little (and even sometimes not so little) mistakes, the irrationalities that kept hitting me in the face as I tried to wend my way through a system that seemed seldom to be humane exacerbated the preoccupation. The angel of death looming over me certainly added to my general irritability and criticality. On the other hand, a focus on the wackiness and meanness of the system and a constant vigilance to make sure that I got what I needed helped me stay on course. And, maybe most important, I maintained a commitment to continue to live my life, do what I always did: I traveled, went to movies and theater, saw friends and family, read books, kept up with *The New Yorker*, enjoyed my grandchildren, did *The Times* Sunday crossword puzzle, celebrated birthdays and anniversaries, went to my Italian class, and played with *Photoshop*—out of breath, sleepy, feeling sick, in pain perhaps; but it never occurred to me to do otherwise.

We all know that aging is a health hazard. Very much like cars, as we get older, systems break down and they don't bounce back as they used to. There is, therefore, abundant reason to assume that my experience has not been very different from that of many people my age: just listen to conversations that older people have—really listen! And for that reason, now that my medical stuff has calmed down or at least feels more under control, I think it might be worthwhile to review some of the events of these last twelve years of mine.

People with terrible diagnoses feel alone and are often alienated from the society just outside their doors! People with cancer are terrified. Elderly people, sick people will have, perhaps, a shock of recognition in what I am about to describe and might profit from my experience, if only by knowing that their experiences within the medical system and their reactions to those experiences are not entirely unique, that they are not alone with their diagnoses, with the callous, patronizing medical attitudes they sometimes experience, and with their often non-verbalized, unarticulated fears. Fears that lie unformulated and unnamed are bitter indeed.

Everybody loves happy endings and, in truth, this is a very happy story: the fact that I have kept surviving, over and over again, that I'm still here, that I thrive, might lift the spirits of those who worry about their own survival. Miracles, as you will see, do, in fact, happen. But for me, the most cogent lesson to be learned from my saga is that you have to take charge of the miracles yourself. The subject of this story is not so much the medical problems that I developed; rather my medical problems are the frame upon which I observe current medical practice.

I

*In which I, a man healthy until this moment,
whose background is herein described, am bestowed
three medical diagnoses,
two of which I know to be fatal*

It had been increasingly a source of pride for me that still, in my late sixties, I was a healthy man, healthier by far than almost everybody I knew: I'd never been in a hospital overnight, I retired from my job with seven months of sick-leave accumulated, on forms I always rated my health as excellent, I was full of energy, and I was frequently told that I looked good. I saw my doctor, Richard Caplin, just once a year. My only contact with Richard was for annual physicals; there was never reason to see him at other times—although we did bump into him at concerts now and then. During the ten years I'd been seeing Richard, there was always mutual respect and we clearly liked each other. I liked the low-keyed way he practiced medicine with me, prescribing drugs only when necessary, respecting my judgment and never patronizing me. His interests were broad and he shared them. He was not only witty himself, but he caught my jokes. All in all, not a bad basis, I feel, for a patient-doctor relationship. I noticed him once across the room at the funeral of a mutual friend, outside of the milieu where I usually saw him, a good-looking man, an imposing,

1

rather elegant figure in his Burberry trench coat. He looked to me like the doctor whom I would choose should look.

I had some minor medical problems, to be sure: like my father, brother, and most men in my family, Dupuytrens Contractures, especially in my left hand (fascia grows on the tendons in the palm of the hand and in the fingers, the muscles contract, and the fingers bend permanently), like my mother, symptoms of Raynaud's disease in both hands (when it's cold, the small arteries in the fingers go into spasm, fingers get numb and turn blue briefly), like no one else in my family, a history of spinal disk problems (which were causing me fewer problems now than they had twenty-five years before), and the assorted aches and pains that come along with living and aging. But these were all minor issues in my general scheme of things and they certainly never got in the way of my doing whatever I wanted to do. The biggest inconvenience that resulted from these minor health problems is that, actually, because of the contractures, I have to wear my wedding ring on my right hand—hardly a sacrifice, I daresay. My point is that I was simply never what I thought of as sick

So, in November 1998, when Richard calls a few days after a routine annual visit (during which each of us comment that I seem to be, as usual, in excellent health) to ask me to go back to the lab to repeat blood tests, I am not at all concerned—not even when he tells me that my white count is a little high. I don't even question the word *little* and I figure that, well, maybe I'd had a *little* cold; I know that there is an increase in white cells when there is a need to fight off infections. My wife, Diana, and I had just come back from the East Coast where we had participated in festivities celebrating Diana's Aunt Betty's ninetieth birthday; the aunt wore heels, she danced with her brother,

her current mah-jongg and bridge friends were guests at the party, and I was convinced, watching her, that there was reason to expect that I too would live forever.

The day after the second lab visit, Richard calls to ask me to come into the office, because, on this repeated blood test, the white count has increased, he says, from about 50,000 to just over 60,000. I have no reference for the numbers themselves—all I know is that my white count was high; surely not too serious, because I know I was a healthy man and Aunt Betty is ninety.

Next day, Diana and I go in and he sees us right away. It is all very awkward, Richard is somewhat more somber than usual, puzzled, and clearly concerned—shrink that I am, I want to help him out, to give him reassurance—and the plan we are able to come up with is that Diana and I will walk on over to see Ernie Rosenbaum, whom Richard calls immediately and who says that he will have room to see me right then. Ernie was the oncologist who had treated Bill, Diana's late husband, for the breast cancer he eventually died from. Ernie and his wife had continued on a friendly basis with Diana. He was sometimes in the columns as oncologist to those who appeared in the columns, and I know from Diana that he spends a lot of evenings at the Opera. I expect from all that I knew about him (except, of course, for the fact of Bill's death, which is a problem for me and keeps me a bit on my toes with him) that he will most probably do right by us. That I am about to see an oncologist, however, and the immediacy of the appointment somewhat startles me, but we are in the neighborhood anyway, so at least the economics are there.

Ernie's office is located two blocks from Richard's, in a building specifically designated for people with cancer, over the entrance, in unmistakable letters, it says, in fact, bold as can be, *Cancer Center*, and I am reluctant to see myself or be seen by others as a *patient* in that facility, my idea being that once you are a patient in a cancer facility, you are indeed a patient in a cancer facility, with all that that implies. We all know the power of labeling. But I am willing to weigh that reluctance against what seems like a rational need, so we go in and, as he said, Ernie is able to see us immediately. I am grateful that we don't have to wait, because the waiting area, well furnished, too large, monochromatic, silent, and completely empty of people, is somehow oppressive and, for me, although well lighted, spooky. We do a lot of social chit-chat in his office, his wife, who runs the office, drops in, it is all very pleasant, but, with all the pleasantries, no one ever forgets for a minute the sub-text of every exchange, our very serious agenda.

He says that, all in all, it looks like some kind of leukemia (LEUKEMIA!!! holy shit! what am I going to do? that's what dying people have! that's what dead people had!), but that there will have to be corroboration from a bone marrow biopsy, which he says he might as well do right then. (What does it mean that everything's happening immediately? Can't we wait a few days? Will I die if we don't do it right now? Or is it that we might as well get this done and out of the way quickly, so we can develop some strategy? Beats me.)

In a bone marrow aspiration and biopsy, I lie on my side or on my stomach, my pants are lowered a few inches, they clean the area where they are going to do the procedure, inject a little something like Xylocaine so it doesn't hurt, a small incision is made over the hip bone in back (the iliac crest to be technical), they rotate a needle back and forth until the bone is penetrated (all I feel is pressure), then they aspirate a little bone marrow; in the biopsy part, they cut a little specimen of the marrow (again I don't feel anything!); essentially, one is liquid, the other solid.

Fortunately for me, unlike many other people, it turns out that this procedure simply doesn't hurt me, it doesn't bother me, I don't have any pain from it. (A very lucky thing for me, since, you will note as you read further, these procedures become routine for me.) That the biopsy isn't particularly uncomfortable, that my pants, though unbuttoned and lowered some, are mostly on, that Diana remains in the office, and that she and Ernie are involved in small talk during the procedure are all very reassuring to me. Somehow I take the informality to signify a situation more benign than it might otherwise be interpreted. He says that he will send the samples off immediately to New Mexico (New Mexico! I even think I understand him to say that this place in New Mexico is the only place that does this kind of analysis, but, given my situation, who knows what he really says) and that we will know for sure in a week whether the problem is indeed Chronic Myelogenous Leukemia as he suspects (*chronic*—as opposed to something *acute*—sounds a little less ominous, a little less terrifying, to me; for me, it means something that you adjust to and that stays around for a very long time; but still, LEUKEMIA! Oh Christ!); he talks about something called the *Philadelphia chromosome*, but, at that point, little registers.

He says that I ought to have a CT Scan just in case his diagnosis of leukemia is not correct and just in case something else is involved and, before I can process what he is saying and be concerned about this *something else*, he is on the phone to set up the scan immediately. Though I am distressed enough with this *chronic* thing, I am beginning to deal with that notion somewhat and I don't want to have to assume the possible burden of *something else*; ambiguity in medical diagnoses doesn't feel good to anyone, I am sure. On the other hand, "Please, let it be leukemia," is not a prayer that conventional wisdom would usually support. Emotional turmoil notwithstanding, Diana and I cross the street dutifully, but numbly, and proceed to Radiology. We don't seem to have other choices.

The CT scanner also sees us right away for the scan; I drink what they give me, I get onto the table (hop doesn't quite express what I do, but I do like the image and, in fact, for a fellow my age, it is sprightly, pretty close to hopping), a rather small and quite attractive young woman comes in, she introduces herself as the radiologist, she injects, she leaves the room, things start moving, terribly loud noises like crashes happen, a disembodied voice (all of a sudden, shades of *Wizard of Oz*) tells me when to hold my breath, when not to move, I keep my eyes shut in order to avoid any visual stimuli that might engender claustrophobia, and finally it is over and I am enormously relieved, mostly that it ended before the eruption of panic and hysteria that seemed imminent to me all the time that I was on the table.

We go back to Ernie's office and he calls the radiologist immediately to ask her impressions. (Perhaps you've noticed that we're getting into doctor's offices and diagnostic procedures without having to wait at all? And we're getting the responsible people on the phone immediately! All we have to do is appear or call! How come, then, when I call on my own to speak with a doctor, getting hold of him/her is a prolonged, frustrating, and sometimes a futile experience?) She says she'll get right back to him, he says something about wet and dry readings, and she very quickly does call back.

Ernie's face looks like he is trying to keep it expressionless as he listens, and then he hangs up and says that a hiatal hernia showed up (here's what a hiatal hernia is: the esophagus and the stomach meet at the diaphragm; that point in the diaphragm, that hole, is called the hiatus; in the case of a hiatal hernia, the stomach bulges a little through the hiatus; that bulge allows stomach acid to get back to the esophagus: that is called acid reflux), that nothing negates the leukemia, and then he adds, with what seems like an attempt at nonchalance, that the radiologist found what looks like a tumor in my left kidney. (A tumor in my left kidney! There went my goddamn future!) Two separate kinds of cancers and the hernia to boot! Wow! I try to be a good citizen, I vote, I do the right thing, I go for an annual visit to my doctor like I'm supposed to, a healthy man, I feel good on arrival, and when I leave, here I am, cancer ridden, and a physical wreck.) The image of Bette Davis doing that thing with the curtains near the end of *Dark Victory* looms large.

The first time I saw Richard Caplin, when he congratulated me for having stopped smoking the year before, I, unable or maybe unwilling (as I still am after twenty three years of abstinence) to release myself from my essential self-concept as a smoker, responded that, "As soon as I get a fatal disease I'm going to start smoking again, and I can't wait." Well, I now have two; should I run out and buy a carton of Pall Malls? Could the smoking option still be there for me? No. I don't think so, and in a way that is too bad: I never had a cigarette I didn't love and I ache still to be near smokers huddled outside office buildings. I guess maybe serious carelessness dissipates some over time.

Now before I go on with the story, I need to make it clear to you that I am not a medical naïf. I have to do that

7

before I can bring you along on this review of my medical experiences over the last twelve years, because I need you to understand that the events that follow do not come about from any lack of sophistication and understanding; that, in truth, I was appealing to and confronting a system I knew well. So I'll begin by telling you something about my past connection to and understanding of how doctors and hospitals operate.

Medical institutions have been a familiar and important part of my adult life. For fifteen years, beginning in 1964, I was full-time faculty at a large medical center and that routinely gave me access to the medical establishment, its mores and thinking—as a matter of fact, I was, a voting member of the medical establishment: for a number of years, for example, I served on the Executive Committee of the College of Medicine.

A psychologist, I supervised medical students in their psychiatric rotation and also was involved in the construction and execution of a course for first year students in how to talk and listen (especially listen) to patients. I taught psychiatric residents and supervised some of their clinical work. I was on a variety of medical school and medical center committees that dealt with such things as the care of medical records, refinement of the delivery of out-patient services, and the responsibility for medical care to the community surrounding the center. For six years on the medical school admissions committee, for example, in conversations and deliberations there about attractive and not attractive attributes of medical school applicants, it was hard to miss medical values and prejudices. I was involved with doctors all the time during those fifteen years, learned how they thought, what they did, and how they operated. In those areas where we had joint projects, there had to

8

be mutual openness between faculty physicians and me, in order to get things done.

I ran a large outpatient psychiatric clinic and was responsible too for what went on in our small inpatient unit. Patients were seen by psychiatric residents, clinical psychology trainees, and social work students, as well as by faculty in all disciplines—but ultimately the responsibility was mine and I had to keep tabs. In addition, I always had a caseload of patients in the clinic and also in a private practice, so I have always been in the mix: I know from a variety of vantage points the complexity of the *doctor* role, how a patient is perceived in both an independent practice and in a complex medical center, and the symbiosis that exists between practitioner and patient. I know too the discomfort in meeting the eyes of frightened clients or patients—it's the price of connecting.

My late wife Sandra was diagnosed with Hodgkin's Disease when she was twenty-three, pregnant with our second daughter, Ruthie. During the next twenty-two years (she died in 1982 at the age of forty-five), we raised our two daughters, we both worked, she went to school, got advanced degrees, taught at a university, was involved in theater; that is, we lived reasonably productive lives, which were sometimes briefly interrupted by recurrences of the disease and by a variety of more or less traumatic kinds of treatments. We always tried to keep on top of what was going on with her and her disease by establishing an easy, open relationship with her doctors, talking at length with all the doctors involved with her over the years and, of course, with my co-faculty members at the medical school, for anything they remembered or recently may have picked up that helped us understand what we ought to think about whatever might be going on with her. In

9

relation to the doctors who treated her, it is likely that, since we were young, rather bright, articulate, open, well educated, and reasonably attractive, that is, people pretty much like themselves (or their children), they treated us in a quite friendly, collegial manner and with some degree of empathy and even surprising openness. So, from two vantage points, from both sides of the desk, I've known my way around hospitals and medical systems fairly well.

My wife Diana had been married to Bill, a psychiatrist, for twenty-two years, until his death in 1978. She was married to him during his internship, residency, and a significant number of years of practice, so hospitals and doctors of all specialties were an every-day part of her life too. And during the last five years of Bill's life, following his cancer diagnosis, there was a good deal of medical and surgical intervention, and, especially because he was a rather young man (forty eight when he died) and a physician to boot, the doctors he dealt with were, of course, very available, both to him and to Diana.

The effect of all these experiences is, I think, exponential. It's unlikely that anybody might consider either of us naïve consumers of medical services. In theory, we know how the system works and even how to work the system. Nothing should get in our way.

And now we begin.

II

In which I learn more about my diagnoses, and am prescribed drugs for one and surgery is scheduled for another.

In dealing with doctors these days, you have to be grateful that they are candid about diagnoses and, from many incidents I know about, however difficult it may be, they try to be honest about prognoses. It wasn't always like this. Let me tell you a little story. Sandra is admitted to the hospital to deliver Annie, our older daughter, and on a routine admissions chest X-ray (that's what they did in those days), they find a "lemon sized" lesion (are you too charmed by the fruit analogies?) in her chest. Many tests later, they still don't know what it is, but we are supposed to watch it. (Imagine having to watch, i.e., do nothing about something in your chest the size of a lemon! In retrospect, it's unbelievable that this is what is asked of a twenty-one year old with a newborn. There is an expectation here, is there not, of accepting something alien as part of you, like in *Invasion of the Body Snatchers*).

Two years later, in the fifth month of Sandra's pregnancy with Ruthie, the obstetrician notices some swelling in her neck, and, given her history, decides on a chest x-ray, which now shows a pineapple sized lesion (again the fruit! but a pineapple now! My God!) in her chest. If these fruit sizes are standard, this thing sure has grown in a couple of years! How do you breathe with something that size in your chest? Because we are stopping in Boston for a month to visit my parents on our way to settling in Chicago, the obstetrician advises a work-up at the Leahy Clinic there.

So in Boston she goes through a lot of tests, some grueling, but, of course, when the evaluation is finished, the clinic refuses to give us any information at all (their lips are sealed despite the fact that we, or our insurance, are paying for the goddamn work-up; the whole thing is, after all, about her and of some considerable consequence to us!); they are willing to speak only to doctors (and to my mother, who does not get off the phone until they tell her, while refusing to give her a diagnosis, that yes, it is serious, and yes, there is good reason to worry; imagine the consequences of that little communication on our family).

We get to Chicago, where we are settling, and Sandra goes to see the radiologist the Leahy Clinic referred her to. He tells her that there is no real concern, but that the day after the baby is born, only for cosmetic purposes, of course, she will start daily radiation to get rid of the rather obviously swollen lymph glands in her neck. It's hard to believe that anyone would fall for that, but she is only twenty-three and about to have a second baby. On the advice of friends, I call him and he asks me to come in. Once I get there, he tells me that the diagnosis is Hodgkin's Disease. I've heard of it, but know nothing about it, except that it's one of those very serious diseases that you know is a very very bad thing to have. I must have paled, because he says, "I have a patient who has lived now twelve years with this disease." To me, at that moment, what he is saying is that if we're very lucky she'll live till she's thirty three years old (the symptoms first showed up two years before) and when she dies, my kids will be motherless at ages ten and twelve. And the fact that he tells me about this woman who lived twelve years with the diagnosis must mean that that is like a record among his patients! Oh, my God!

I'm in a panic! I'm thinking about how I'm going to talk about this with Sandra, how are we going to deal with this (Christ! She's only twenty-three! How am I going to lay the burden of this diagnosis on her? What will I do if she dies? How can I lose her? My kids—orphans! Aren't you supposed to be older to deal with problems like this! This happens to people of my parents' generation!), but he says that we should not tell her the diagnosis (and certainly not the prognosis, I suppose—not even if I let her know about his patient who lived twelve years; apparently now that has stopped sounding so swell to him too), because she needs all her strength and morale: she is very young, he explains, in her eighth month of pregnancy, with a two year old at home. I argue that I don't think I can do that, I don't like dishonesty, it will create problems between her and me, I need to tell her the truth, and we need somehow to deal with this together.

But he is absolutely certain about the right thing to do, he is adamant and he pushes and pushes, I'm twenty-nine, he's head of his department, elderly, sophisticated, and experienced in the world (he goes to Dubrovnik on vacations), so I finally agree. I go back to work, my head whirling, my heart breaking, and once back in my office, I find my Merck Manual (gathering dust until this moment), and look up Hodgkin's Disease (this is 1960); it begins: "Hodgkin's Disease is a fatal disease . . . . " I close the book.

Ruthie is born and, beginning the following day, Sandra shows up (she is wheeled from Maternity down to Radiation

Therapy in the basement) for daily radiation, (which, by the way is, sufficiently primitive at that time, that the scarring in her lungs is the basis for serious problems later). I'm at work one day about a month into the radiation series, the phone rings, and Sandra asks me, "What is Hodgkin's Disease?" Insurance forms had come, and on them, clear as could be, was the diagnosis. In the course of the conversation, she realizes that I've been aware of the diagnosis, assumes that the concealment—the lie—was in order to prevent her from knowing that death is imminent and she assumes also that I cannot be trusted—or at least she wonders how she is to know if any statements about her physical condition are honest or lies. Although this all gets worked out after a while, while it lasts it is not good for anybody—certainly not for Sandra—except maybe for the radiologist.

I am sure that you will agree that the moral of this story clearly is that secrets in a family do damage. But what did we really learn from this experience? In practice, I'm afraid, nothing. Ruthie is a newborn and Annie is two. I want this condition of Sandra's to be an open issue, certainly within the family. I want the children, as they grow, to know pretty much what is going on with their mother and thus not be frightened by silence and secrets and then later by the name of the disease. I don't want secrets. Sandra feels that they (at any age, it seems) are too young to have to deal with the anxiety connected with her diagnosis (this seems to be precisely what her doctor said to me in relation to Sandra's knowing, isn't it! From my point of view, this is identification with the oppressor). We have many discussions over the years, and I feel that I can't go against her wishes—it is, after all, her disease!

So we say almost nothing to the children and each time there is a recurrence or any other problem connected with the disease, we light-pedal to them what's going on with their mother, give it no name, and offer no explanation. There is a humongous elephant in the living room and no one can mention it. This has to have some serious effect on the kids growing up; and when they learn the truth, what will be the meaning of this secrecy to them? It is a quagmire for me. And then, when they are eleven and thirteen and Sandra is going through some kind of treatment, I finally prevail on her and we discuss her Hodgkin's Disease with the children. But I think the damage is long done.

One more story, a quickie this time, and then, I promise, we'll get on with my own spine-tingling saga. My brother calls late spring the year my kids are ten and twelve to say that the illness that has my father down has been diagnosed, unfortunately, as pancreatic cancer. I say that we are going to England and will stop in Boston for a few days on the way, to check things out, and we do. In the car, bringing us from the airport, my brother tells me that my mother is not to know what my father's diagnosis is. Here we go again!

The implicit message here is that my father also should not know, but I can take on only one thing at a time. I say, "Do you think she doesn't notice that he's sick, debilitated, and being treated by doctors? She's going to find out that he died when he dies. They are married and have been together for forty-four years! Why hide it now?" Mind you, my mother, though prone to hysteria, is a sophisticated, knowing woman—she reads the newspaper every day, she reads contemporary novels, she is aware of what is going on in the world. How can one not tell her? My brother is resolute and so apparently are all my relatives and the entire staff of Boston's Beth Israel Hospital; so, not a word to my mother.

15

We go to England, our first trip abroad together, come back, have a little summer, and then, after Labor Day, my brother calls to tell us that my father is back in the hospital, he is very sick, he seems terminal. We fly to Boston, all of us, and stop at the hospital on the way to my parents' apartment. Sandra and I go up to see my father (the kids, ages ten and twelve are not allowed to visit in patient areas, so they wait in the lobby, with the result that my father does not see his grandchildren, nor they their sweet and loving grandfather). My father dies during the night, my brother and I go to the hospital early in the morning for whatever business has to be done there and when I come back, my mother asks me, "Tell me the truth, Paul. Did he have cancer?" What a pathetic situation for a mourning widow to be in, asking her son what it was that her husband has been suffering with for months and that had just killed him! And what the hell was my father supposed to be thinking those last weeks, literally on his deathbed?

Now let's get back to my story. Ernie sets up appointments for me to be seen a few days later, first in the hematology clinic by a leukemia maven and then one hour later and one floor higher by the big kidney surgery. Diana and I are early for the hematology appointment (notice that I don't call it *oncology*? Do you think that that might give a hint about how I deal with illness? Stay tuned!). Walking into the waiting area, seeing my co-patients, now my brothers, is quite a push to reality! A nurse takes us to an office that seems in no way to be an office; there are no walls and it is, rather, a part of the corridor and secluded from nothing.

The nurse, strangely distracted (it might be contact lenses or maybe even a post-nasal drip) and seemingly anxious, interviews me about my demographics, my symptoms (there are none!), and my recent medical history about which there is very little to say. I mention that we have an appointment with the kidney surgeon in an hour, she becomes even more nervous, says that that cannot be, because this oncology appointment is to last two hours. Although she calls the kidney surgeon's office to change our appointment to an hour later, whether or not this gets agreed to at the other end remains unclear to us because this nurse speaks always ambiguously and somehow it's hard to get her to make her statements, even about this appointment, more definite.

When this rather eccentric, but very brief encounter is over, she takes us to the person who is going to weigh me and record vital signs—such a lovely and even dramatic name for such pedestrian things: blood pressure, pulse, temperature, and respiration. When that procedure is done, I am to wait until called by the lab people for blood work. The waiting area is actually a wide corridor, all windows on one side, offering one of the more dramatic views in the city—any tourist can identify San Francisco from that view and any patient, not completely crazed with and turned completely off by anxiety, swells up with pride at the beauty of the view. Against both walls are lined up unmatched chairs, and, on the window side, there is a small table with two large thermos carafes, one with brewed coffee, the other with hot water, a stack of paper (not Styrofoam) cups, a plastic basket holding tea bags in foil, packets of real and fake sugar, a jar of fake powdered cream, and a paper plate holding a few sad boughten cookies.

After what is actually a short wait, but one that seems interminable to me (because at that point, what wouldn't seem interminable to me? and because, despite how well I feel, up and down the waiting area are people with cancer, very pale, ashen, pitifully thin, fragile looking people, people with almost transparent skin, women with head scarves or turbans, very young bald men, boys really, people who need help to walk, people with shunts—and yet the area is full of sounds of joking and banter and, of course, foot traffic to and from the coffee set-up, all of them, all of us, trying to act as though the situation is a normal one—all in all, a very potent suggestion to me of what will very likely be my experience shortly down the line!), my name is called, blood is drawn, and we sit again. After maybe twenty minutes we are taken to a small examining room and told that the doctor—Charlie Linker is how Ernie had referred to him—will be in soon and in a very short time he enters.

What I notice immediately about this man who, to my thinking, is to be my savior—he is, after all, going to cure me of something that is, without him, going to be terrible—is that he is wearing a very nice shirt, has great cheekbones and very impressive graying hair; he seems open, straightforward, and engaged. For me, at that moment, these attributes are very important and make up for the lousy old magazines in the waiting area: my salvation depends completely on my liking this fellow and so far he has won me. I mean, if he's not what I consider a good guy, then he surely won't be able to do me good. (Logical? That is not the point. I'm desperate and it's the way I think.) And after he introduces himself, there is a short exchange, and then he says, "Ernie Rosenbaum said that it looks like you have acute myelogenous leukemia."

Very quickly, in order to prevent any paranoia about Ernie developing in me and to stave off any overt, shared dread about my life expectancy, I say with as much calm as I can bring to bear, "No, no, no. He told us that he thought it was chronic." "Oh," says Charlie, "excuse me a minute" and he leaves the room. So what's going to happen to me now that I am in the hands of someone who not only doesn't read the referral or remember what was said, but expects the worst! I need an optimist! They give you hope, these guys, and then, when you least expect it, pull it away. I am dead!

Let me take a few minutes here to give you some facts about Chronic Myelogenous Leukemia. First, let's refer to it henceforth as CML. I'm going to try to make this as non-Merck Manual as I can, but I think it's helpful to know what it is we are following. Leukemia is a blood cancer, but instead of tumors, there is an overproduction of white cells; the name *leukemia,* comes from the Greek words for *white* and *blood*. The proliferation of white cells in the bone marrow ultimately gets in the way of red blood cell production and the production of platelets, leading to anemia and also a lack of proper clotting, for starters.

Leukemia can be acute or chronic, lymphocytic or myelogenous (called myelogenous or myeloid because the while cells contain tiny granules). We are concerned here only with the chronic myelogenous kind (again, CML), and because I know nothing about them and don't want to bore you, I'll skip the others, except for one thing: chronic myelogenous is rather aggressive and escalates (the amount of time in this escalation varies) to an acute phase; and then, after a while, it is, as they say, curtains.

They don't know quite what causes leukemia, but there are hunches that point to such things as radiation (lots of leukemia in Hiroshima after the bomb, remember?) and maybe even, for example, smoking: for me, not much radiation, as far as I know, but lots of unfiltered Pall Mall cigarettes until ten years before my diagnosis. (It seems to me unlikely that it would it be those fluoroscope things in shoe stores when I was a kid; they were there for mothers to check out the fit of the prospective purchase on their children's feet, but it was used by the children to check out their foot bones and to watch their toes wiggle—unlikely, because, if that were the primary source, CML would not be so rare an occurrence.) In CML, chromosomes develop an anomaly, which is called the Philadelphia Chromosome (named for the City of Brotherly Love, where the finding about this anomaly was made). Human DNA has twenty=three pair of chromosomes. In people with CML, chromosomes 9 and 22 interchange a piece, and this produces an abnormal gene (it's called BCR-ABL), which, in turn, produces an abnormal protein (Bcr-Abl tyrosine kinase) and it is this protein that causes the proliferation of white cells. (This is as technical as I'm going to get, I promise.). Oh, by the way, it is important to make clear that this chromosomal abnormality, this mutation, is not innate and is not passed on. It is an acquired mutation, and hence, as I mentioned, the issues of such things as radiation and smoking.

Maybe it's the strange interchange between chromosomes that accounts for the fact that there are relatively few cases of this disease—fewer than five thousand new cases a year in this country. That there are so few (and five thousand is actually a small number of people; consider, for example, the enormous number of new diabetes and breast cancer cases each year—a million and a third adults and two hundred thousand women respectively) makes it now relatively unprofitable for a drug company to spend a lot of money developing and marketing a drug that so few people will be buying. The expected income from sales of the drug, because the disease is so infrequent, is simply not worth the huge outlay of money that R&D on a new drug requires. OK. You get the picture of what I've got and what it's going to do. Now on with me.

So in a matter of minutes Charlie returns and says, "You're right! The good news is that you have *Chronic* Myelogenous Leukemia; the bad news is that you have leukemia," and he goes into a discussion about leukemia. He tells us what the Philadelphia chromosome is and assures us that the findings are back from New Mexico and validate the diagnosis. He says that the only real, for certain, cure for this disease is a bone marrow transplant, but, first of all, the donor has to be a perfect match (anyway, we find out later, that my brother, my only sibling, who, as soon as he heard my diagnosis, volunteered his marrow, turns out to be not even close to a perfect match—and it's next to impossible to find anyone besides a sibling—his/her genes come from the same sources that mine do; nobody else then has as high a probability of having DNA like mine—who will even come close) and secondly, the survival rate for a bone-marrow transplant in people my age, even with an ideal donor is less than fifty percent. Need I tell you, this gives me pause, indeed. We must be talking about something very serious here! And the only real cure cannot be available to me!

He talks about prognosis: if I'm not one of the small minority to get rid of the Philadelphia chromosome on Hydroxyurea, a drug he is about to prescribe for me, or Interferon, which he will prescribe later if the Hydroxyurea does not work after a certain number of months to get rid of the Philadelphia chromosome, life expectancy is three to ten years. I simply know, I know for certain, there is no doubt whatsoever in my mind, I must believe that one of these drugs will completely wipe away my disease; three to ten years is simply not time enough; but I do know also that in my case, if the drugs, by some remote chance, don't work, it's going to be closer to ten years for me than to three, and in those ten years God knows what they will come up with. I won't have it otherwise. We chat, everything is cool, I like him now. (i.e., my life expectancy has just increased). He answers all our questions very candidly and with clarity; there is no talking down to us, no skirting possibilities. Our conversation is running down, it's time to leave, he gives me a prescription and an appointment to return in a week, and I say with complete confidence, "I want you to understand. Have no doubt. I am going to beat this mother-fucker," and we leave.

I need to add a comment here. Sandra died mid-September 1982 and was dying all that summer. I knew that, so long as I insisted that she was going to live, she would live, and I, therefore, exerted a lot of energy to convince myself and family and friends that she really wasn't that sick, that of course she was going to make it. Denial, a defense mechanism that I battled against in psychotherapy patients during my professional career, became a chronic and necessary way of life for me. Those who visited her in the hospital after speaking with me were certainly in for a surprise. I want you to understand that logically I never really thought I had the power to keep her alive, but at a level beneath or beyond logic I prohibited myself from looking at her situation realistically, because negative consequences to her might then ensue; it was more like if she became aware that I thought she was dying, she would give up the ghost and die.

This point of view can result in some very strange and stupid, even destructive behavior: my brother tells me on the phone that he wants to fly out to see Sandra, I, feeling that if she sees him, having flown across the country, she will correctly interpret his flying this far to see her, especially without his wife, to mean that she is dying, so I beg him not to come; what is it with him? doesn't he remember that our father died the night of the day that Sandra and I flew out to see him? doesn't he understand the connection? He comes though, and, insanely, I do not allow him to see her, and I continue to suffer the consequences of this stupidity of mine even now. Did I know she was dying? Of course! But I couldn't let on that that was true and had to insist, certainly to her, but even to myself that she would live. The power, of course, of magical thinking and omnipotence is, however, very limited and reality is, without any doubt, going to overwhelm it, so when she does in fact die, no one is really caught off guard. Well, it's the same business here.

I know pretty well what the mortality from my new disease is (I listen and read well enough), and unless I affirm my power over it, it's going to get me. So I automatically force myself to believe and push to convince everyone that I'm in contact with to understand, that I am stronger than this son of a bitch and it's not going to get me, it will not kill me! "It's no big deal," I communicate; in retrospect, given the names of these conditions of mine, these people must have thought I was crazy; that leukemia and kidney cancer (or better still, renal cell carcinoma) are "no big deal" is quite a stretch. But I'll use anything. Essentially it's like bluffing in poker: as long as "they" believe you, you're going to win, you're going to live. Of course I know that this is nonsense, but, whatever the logic, better to fight than to lie back and give in.

Now back to the events. Out of the area, buoyed by Charlie's candor and unwillingness to patronize, we are

23

pleased to notice that there's still time to keep the original appointment with the kidney surgeon. That means that what was supposed to take two hours, however long it seemed, took only one hour; my life is determined in a one-hour shot! But still, it seems a good omen and so far we don't have much else to go by but omens. Despite my obsessing about the fact that we should take the stairs instead of an elevator to go up only one flight of stairs, in view of our not being able to find the stairs, we ride up the one floor, find our way to the office, and they tell us that the doctor is in surgery, but will be sure to call us later in the day. It was less than an hour ago that the nurse had changed the appointment. Does this man wait for any excuse to run to surgery? Don't they still schedule operations in advance? What would have happened to the person being operated on right this minute if our appointment hadn't been fouled up? But the situation at least gives us the opportunity to return home now, needing to minimize only one of my two conditions and we can still ignore the other; for me, for all practical purposes right now, the kidney tumor is not real.

Alas, however, soon after we get home, he calls (like he ran directly from the OR to a phone); he says that yes, he's gotten all the material, yes, there is indeed a tumor in my left kidney, and we should come in to discuss what ought to be done about it. We set up the appointment, although my impulse is to continue to ignore the kidney for the time being and focus all my attention on the leukemia. It's hard enough to work denial or even something constructive on one process; on two it seems impossible. My reasoning, at that moment, is that only if I can feel in control of the disease can I get rid of it and it takes a certain amount of energy to convince at least myself that I have some control in one area. OK, so now he says the kidney tumor is real, but I insist to myself that it's very likely been there for years, is not growing, is not malignant, and thus, in fact, I don't really need a kidney surgeon.

Nevertheless we go to the appointment. I do not allow my now ubiquitous, but rather flimsy, brittle denial system to intrude too directly, too certainly, on reality, and we go. But once there, how do you deal with a young man (he seems younger than he should), oozing charm, smiling, full of energy, light-pedaling, joking, wearing a patterned shirt with a white collar, when one is facing a death sentence and he holds your life in his hands? I resent not only the collar and the manner, but especially the power he has suddenly usurped from me; the collar and the manner merely afford me concrete targets for my resentment.

He asks very cheerfully if we want to see the CT scan. Actually, I have little interest in seeing the scan, since the ability to read them is not a gift I was born with and I know to rely on experts for diagnoses. There is, however, no opportunity to reject the invitation, he is already running into the next room. We follow him (we, though, walk); the scan is already on the light box, waiting for us. What he points to as a tumor is for me only the barest smudge; no doubt about it, though, I've got to take what he says as fact because he's the expert. He has the arcane and sometimes useful facility to read these things. I am amazed at the amount of information this smudge gives him; but then, I suppose, it's like all the information I used to get out of a Rorschach. It's also like Edward Arnold in either *Eyes in the Night* or *The Hidden Eye*—it was quite a long time ago and I don't remember which: he's a blind detective (the same detective with the same service dog in each movie), hiding in a closet, when a bad guy is making a phone call to the so far unidentified head bad guy; he (Edward) is able

25

to find out who the head bad guy is because he can learn the phone number the lesser bad guy dials by the number of clicks the rotary phone makes. This too is an arcane and useful facility, so long as rotary phones are in use—and one is blind.

Hoping I'm asking the right questions (I want to do well even here!), I talk to him about options (surgery vs. waiting), about probabilities of malignancy (very high), about why not a biopsy (too many false negatives), about the likelihood of removing the tumor and not the kidney (very high), and all the time I'm there, what I really want to do is thank him and get myself and Diana the hell out of there. But we stay! (Again my easily penetrated denial system!)

He says that if, worst-case scenario, the entire kidney has to be removed, it would not be, by any means, a major disaster for me, because the remaining kidney takes over the function of the one removed. (Maybe not a major disaster for him! But he cannot convince me that having only one of two things you're born with and therefore supposed to have is even close to a good deal!). He says that he doesn't think there is an emergency. I ask, if the probability of its being malignant is so high, why isn't it an emergency? Although my question certainly seems direct to me, it may be that somehow it is not direct enough, because he doesn't tell; my question evaporates as though it serves no function, so that even I cannot follow it up.

He says that he wants to make sure that it's all right to do the surgery at this time, given the leukemia and the medicine I'm on, and that he would like me to speak to Charlie about that before he schedules the surgery. I do not suggest to him that it would make more sense for him to speak with Charlie himself, they are, after all, only one floor apart and they do speak the same medical jargon and, in the abstract at least, it sounds better that doctors dealing with supposed disparate parts of me communicate, because isn't there some rhetoric about the *whole* person. And, God knows, using an intermediary (me) is not the most efficient way to communicate. But he has asked me to do it, so I'll do it.

And I'll take advantage of this opportunity! "Great!" I think to myself. "Then we don't have to schedule the surgery or think about this ever again." In my heart of hearts, whatever this man says, I am sure, I have convinced myself that the tumor is benign and has been sitting there forever. So my plan is to put off dealing with it as long as I am able.

It makes sense to mention in this context that my experience and that of many people I have talked to convince me that if you are seeing more than one doctor, especially if they are in different specialties, you are likely in trouble. It seems that doctors not only don't talk to doctors in specialties other than their own, but also they seem not even to read the chart notes or write-ups by people outside their specialties. So if two separate systems of yours that are being treated interact in any way or if drugs in more than one system interact, forget about it. It's likely that nobody will find out and do something about it, unless you talk it up with all of them. You will see how these problems develop with me as you read on.

On our way home, Diana and I talk about the fact that there are people who have to be informed about this situation of mine, of ours—even with my plan to defer dealing with the kidney. The people highest on the list are, of course, my kids, Annie and Ruthie, both in their late thirties (you'll remember that I didn't like keeping them in the dark, at a much younger age, about their mother's health issues). We decide that we'll invite them over of an evening, have like a family meeting, and let them know just what the scoop is. We invite and they arrive.

We sit in the living room, Diana in a rocking chair, I in a side chair opposite Annie, Ruthie, and Ruthie's husband, all three of them on the sofa. When I begin to talk, I can see how distressing the subject of my health is for them and I certainly don't want to cause them any distress. Not only do I hate to see them unhappy, but I sense even more that their distress about my health makes me surprisingly unhappy; in fact, I resent it, it makes me mad. I want them to affirm that my situation is really not something to worry about, because otherwise I'm going to become very anxious myself; there is that little system that I've built up to deal with these things and I can't have their overt worry shooting my defenses down. So I give them the facts, but I soft-pedal everything. Apparently I'm not doing enough soft-pedaling, because they are very quickly in tears and Ruthie's husband is saying to Ruthie, "Now we'll never leave San Francisco for New York," and all I can do is offer more and more reassurance, without lying outright. It's crazy! I have the cancers, but I need to comfort them.

There is clearly something wrong with this picture, but, in fact, I don't know how to make it otherwise. In the midst of their tears, it becomes clear to me that the idea that my two cancers might be connected appeals to them. This makes no sense to me at all, except for the serendipity of our finding out about them at the same time; but, because, for some reason, that possibility makes things a little less horrific for them (I guess it would mean that there is really only one thing wrong with me instead of two; what they might be missing, however, is that one thing can kill as efficiently as two—death happens, in general, only once), I tell them that I'll check about a possible relationship when I go to see the doctors again (I do and they confirm that there is really no relationship) and, *father* that I am, as time goes on, I find myself giving them as much support as I can.

Any time there are untoward results of any kind about anything medical with me, even with my commitment to honesty, I shade the information I give to my kids in a way that is not quite lying, so I can still tell myself that I've been open and honest. So much for disclosure! And in my state yet, I choose to be the supportive agent. Why am I not thinking that they are old enough and competent enough to be doing that job for me? For the next five years, any time I hear that anxiety in their voices, that little choke, that little pause, a question worded in a way that to me reveals a subtext of worry, a suggestion that my medical problems are to be taken seriously, I am very uncomfortable, maybe there is even a twinge of anger, and I need to cool them off or hang up. I do understand that this reassurance of mine distances me from what would be an attack on my denial of the severity of my situation. It does alas, become clearer and clearer, doesn't it, that it's not them I'm worried about, it's me!

The following week we're in to see Charlie. My white count is down appreciably and we all feel nice about that, even though Charlie lets us know that while the drug has indeed lowered the white count, there is no indication that it has affected the disease and its progression at all. But at least something positive is going on. While chatting, he asks us what has happened about my kidney tumor. I can't lie to him. We tell him about our appointment, he says that the leukemia and the medication do not preclude the surgery, I venture that I'm actually in no rush to have the surgery and would like to wait a while and watch the tumor (remember, in my defense, the kidney guy did assure me that this is not an emergency) and he says, clearly with disapproval reverberating, "I wouldn't walk around long with a tumor in my kidney."

Whoops! I cannot afford his disapproval. He's telling me to get this (for me, up until this point, nuisance) tumor taken care of as soon as possible, that cancers do metastasize and kill, and that it's not realistic that I make judgments about things I know nothing about. So now I'm stuck. I can't deny any more: I don't want to die—and Charlie and Diana are, at some level, wise to me. I have to call the kidney surgeon and tell him what Charlie said and, in my now black and white world, put my life back in his hands.

I want to add another comment about his statement. Not only has he been willing here to offer me advice, but he's used himself as a reference. This man is being open with me about himself and about me, and he is a doctor—one of the very few I have known as a patient who is willing to do that. He is putting himself in my shoes and suggesting what he feels is best to do. Pretty close to empathy, I'd say. And he avoids my feeling pushed because he turns it around on himself.

A few days later, there's a return visit to the surgeon and this time, despite his glad-hand and charm, I get the feeling that he doesn't want us to dawdle; I feel patronized by his attitude toward us and by his answers to the few question I muster. Why don't these people know how to talk to people who are as smart as they are? And then he says that, gee, he doesn't seem to have any surgery openings for several weeks. Can you believe this? It's a kind of bait and switch! It's a tease! And now, suddenly, it becomes very clear to me that, instead of applying a little rationality and postponing the procedure a few weeks there is no way I can wait at all.

Now that I've made the decision and taken myself this far, how can this arrogance get in my way! I implore, trying to make it not look like imploring, he calls his secretary out, and suddenly, after conferring *sotto voce* with her, both examining schedules carefully, he announces that he can arrange space the following week—it is almost as though his holding off was intended to make me more eager. But I'm not going to hold grudges nor ask how this scheduling miracle turned up and, instead, we set up a definite date for surgery.

Before leaving the office, I ask about the size and whereabouts of my future incision, of the scar. As soon as the words are out of my mouth, I am aware that he doesn't like the question—there is a nanosecond delay and an extraordinarily transient disapproval in his facial expression, but he regains his usual aplomb and smile, and tells me about several possibilities. Knowing that I am about to offend, that he will not view the eruption of my narcissism with any degree of pleasure, but unable to stop myself, I tell him that I want the smallest scar possible and, while I'm at it, I make sure again that he knows without any doubt that I want only the tumor removed, and that the kidney itself had best stay in my body where it belongs, that only the most dire circumstances, the very last resort, could ever possibly justify the removal of the kidney. At this point, I am sure that he hates me and will do as much damage as he can get away with. But I also know that I'm more than a little nuts and that things will go as well as they can. Ambivalence is not a new experience for me and people often turn out better than I expect them to.

I want you to understand that throughout this saga I am not really, seriously, at this moment, attributing motives to anyone except myself. I am trying to give you a picture of my experience and my perceptions and my fears. The incidents are factual and the quotes are as real as memory allows, but my conjectures about anyone else's motives are a reflection of how I felt, what things meant to me, what the reality around me led me to suppose about the people I was dealing with and I expect that my vulnerability led me just about always to suppose the worst. Feeling lousy physically and being frightened are surely going to color one's perceptions. It is true though that the specifics of how people operate and what they say and don't say do enable one to read into the situation whatever those specifics allow—there is always room for some personal interpretation, tone of voice, blink of eye, any minimal gesture; paranoid people take advantage of situations into which they can easily knit their perhaps personal thinking, but so also, though in a less spectacular way, do people without psychiatric diagnoses.

I have no doubt that my personal needs and my personality attributes play a large part in the organization of my perception of events. Something happens that many other people might let slide and for them it fades away, while for me the event might insinuate itself into brilliant focus and, of course, vice versa—I might pass over things that might preoccupy some other people. Nevertheless, the event did occur; something happened, it can be photographed or taped—it is its significance, what it means, that may be up for grabs.

Let me use a psychotherapy analogy. In orthodox psychoanalytic psychotherapy, the crux is in the analysis of the transference, but every psychoanalytic therapist knows that he has to keep his eye on who he is and what he communicates to the patient and how that stimulates responses to him by the patient. It isn't quite kosher to think that the patient is projecting his thing onto a blank screen; there really is another person in the room and, however much he tries to be neutral, it is impossible not to be communicating cues about himself, his mood, his state of health, his reactions, etc. It's like that here. However distorted, however exaggerated, however personal, however off-the-wall my thinking is about these people I'm dealing with, there is something about them, something they communicate, that I am reacting to. As our old sages and marital counselors used to say, "It takes two to tango."

Now that I know that I'm going to have the surgery, I have to deal with what becomes for me an important issue: I don't own any pajamas, and, since I'm going to stay in the hospital four or five days after the operation, I had better get out and buy some; after all, you do want to look nice. And in fact, it's nicer to think about pajamas, than about somebody cutting you up. In the store, I find that the price of pj's has increased quite a bit since I was in high school when my mother bought me my last pair and I resent spending so much on attire that I will be wearing only a few days. So I go to the sale bin and find a pair of Calvin Klein pajamas on sale, reasonably priced. The problem (and, I figure, the reason that they are on sale) is that the top is short sleeved, the bottoms are like Bermuda shorts, and the stripes are nothing I would choose. There is a clown quality to them, but they do have a Calvin Klein label (even though I alone will know that) and it's only for a few days, so I buy them. It turns out that while in the hospital, given the presence of catheters and tubes, I have to content myself with what the hospital has put me in and I wear the pajamas for a few days after I get home, and then, of course, never again. But

I save them in case a more opportune occasion for such an outfit arises.

Two days before the surgery, I go to the hospital for the required pre-op work-up. When I get to the office to which my papers direct me and show the clerk the papers I'd been given, she tells me that there is an error on the papers, that I'm in the wrong place, that the information, the room number, on the papers is wrong, and that I have to go first to register at a different office, down the hall—the Admissions office—and then return to this one. Am I going overboard to think that that this does not bode well? Now, I know that my being directed to the wrong office is a minor issue, but surely it reveals something about a system that has not corrected the error that clearly has happened to every patient to whom standard papers similar to mine have been given. As the old wisdom has it, "Little things mean a lot."

The order of offices now cleared up, I register in Admissions after a surprisingly short wait, they hand me a file and send me back to where I'd just come from. I, of course, open the file, look at the forms, and see that the surgery scheduled for me is a *radical nephrectomy*. A radical nephrectomy! I know nephrectomy means cutting out a kidney; how can anything be more radical than just a plain conservative nephrectomy? They add the word radical, I think, to make sure that we understand that they are really serious about doing it or is it just to rub it in, to pour salt on my newly acquired wounds? And he had promised that he would remove the kidney only as a last resort. Lying arrogant son of a bitch! His collar should have warned me! It's my body! It is my fucking kidney! He cannot do this to me.

I manage to pull myself together (if only because it would be unseemly for a person of my age and station simply to collapse onto the floor and cry) and call him on a hospital phone that some kind soul allows me to use. I get him in. I ask why the paperwork indicates a radical nephrectomy when he has promised that he will make every effort to remove only the tumor. Quick as a bunny, not missing a beat, he tells me that one has to schedule for the worst possibility in order to reserve enough time in the operating room and that, of course, his aim is to remove only the tumor.

I don't know what to think of this (I still don't). I am close to believing what he says, because after he saw me initially, he wrote a note to Ernie Rosenbaum, the referrer, who sent me a copy, to wit: "I might attempt a partial nephrectomy, given the size and location of the lesion, If the intraoperative frozen section reveals the lesion to be benign, I would proceed with partial nephrectomy. If the lesion is identified to be malignant, but all surgical margins and the rest of the kidney look normal, I would consider renal reconstruction rather than nephrectomy." And, even more, I sort of believe him because his response is so quick, there hasn't been time to think up an excuse; but I am still suspicious, I am paranoid, I am a wild man. To keep the two kidneys I was born with has become a very big thing for me and I know that it's good to be vigilant because sometimes doctors do make mistakes. We read about them in the papers. And here are a couple of personal examples:

> Sandra is at a routine appointment in relation to the Hodgkin's Disease, a follow-up appointment after a series of radiation. Her regular doctor is away (probably sunning again in Dubrovnik), so they assign her a different one for that visit. At that time, each of her two bouts with the disease happened when

she was pregnant. Despite that, this new doctor tells her that she ought to get pregnant, because there was evidence recently published that in women with a history of the disease, pregnancies reduce the probability of recurrence. Well, maybe. But Sandra's records clearly indicate, however, that in her case the reverse is true.

Here's another, very recent:

A close friend with a history of heart problems (angioplasty twelve years ago and completely symptom-free since then) experiences, for a second day, tightness in his chest walking up-hill; he goes to the hospital emergency room, where, at first, his history is taken and, when asked about allergies, he says, "Beta—blockers," the clerk asks what has happened when he has taken them, he says that he stops breathing, she enters the information into the computer, and says that she will prepare a wrist-band to that effect. A few moments later, he is now on a bed in a room in the ER, the wrist-band not yet attached, a nurse comes in, and, in response to his question about what she is doing, says that she is preparing an IV and will soon also be giving him a beta-blocker. Picture the situation had he been sleeping, had he not questioned her, had he simply lain back and trusted the system.

Of course, I can think of a number of other such situations, and if I can think of others, so can you. Multiply these examples across the country and you understand why one had better be on one's toes.

Anyway, I go back to the first office, a little less agitated now, wait my turn, blood is drawn, and they do an EKG. As soon as the EKG is finished, I'm buttoning my shirt, I'm not quite off the table, a woman comes up to me, introduces herself as the admitting physician and asks, with no hemming and hawing, whether I've recently had a heart attack—like I don't have enough to deal with as it is. My kidney surgeon is secretly plotting to remove my kidney and I've just had a heart attack?

I say "What?" pulling together as cool an attitude as I am able to fake (I am really close to passing out), she is puzzled about something relating to the lower left quadrant of my heart, and I tell her that during my annual physical, when all this started, about a month earlier, an EKG was done and actually no heart attack was mentioned. I suggest that she speak directly with Richard about my heart, but that idea doesn't seem to please her—perhaps his not being on the university faculty plays into that displeasure. She is willing though to contact Richard's office, get the month old material, and compare the two.

She goes away and soon is back, saying that, surprisingly, today's EKG looks even better than the one I had the month before, but that we will still have to do a stress test before I am OK'd for anesthesia. This reasoning makes no sense to me—if there were a problem, and, of course, there really isn't (I think Richard would at least have mentioned it and certainly would be open to discuss it with this woman right now), and if it's getting better, one would assume that there is very little to be concerned about—but we all know by now how I tend to minimize and deny, and who am I anyway to dispute her thinking.

I push to get it dealt with right now, to have it over with. Picture this: with all my ambivalence about the surgery I am trying to talk this young woman into allowing it to go ahead. And, in my now ridiculous frame of mind, the sooner the better. Again what I really want is to take advantage of the situation, spring right out of there, run to the airport with Diana and settle down by a beach in Belize, for good, without a phone, without a mailing address—but if we are going to do this goddamn surgery, let's get it done now. Do I define ambivalence here? She gets on the phone and begins to call people who might enable us to get a treadmill stress test done immediately, but everyone's away, out to lunch, full schedule—and perhaps most important, after all, only six more shopping days till Christmas; future appointments are offered, but none in time for an OK for surgery two days thence.

And then, out of the blue someone is available to do it (Why are the right people always the last to be called? Just joking!), not by treadmill, but by using some heart revving-up drug. And so we do it; we go upstairs, there is a rather tight crowd of six of us in the small room, surrounding a monitor, like we're all watching a show—starring . . . in its debut role . . . my heart! (Perhaps you wonder why hospital costs are so high? Could it be because everybody is keeping everyone else company watching such interesting things as my beating heart!) The atmosphere in the room is like that at a screening of what could be an exciting new movie. They hook me up, inject me with the drug, the technician is very friendly and explains throughout what we're looking at, they have positioned me so that I can see the monitor clearly, my heart on the monitor apparently looks dandy to everybody (to me it looks vulnerable and achy, but spirited), so we're on.

The surgery will take place in two days—a Thursday (i.e. two days before the weekend and eight days before Christmas, acceded to without a thought to what this timing might signify about vacations and days off for hospital staff).

III

*In which surgery takes place and I face challenging
adventures while in the hospital*

Two days later, Diana and I arrive at 6:00 AM at the hospital area where we are supposed to be, just as we were instructed (There has to be some reason that this surgical stuff always has to start so early? Who decrees these ungodly hours? Who else is awake at this hour, let alone on the street?—insomniacs and maybe druggies! What do surgeons do the rest of the day? Can't they golf (or whatever else they now do in the afternoon in the morning instead and do their surgery at a more civilized hour?); after a short wait, a woman, elderly, clearly a volunteer, takes us, everyone who has come in at that hour with an appointment for surgery, tired, zombie-like from too little sleep and too much worry, in a group, walking to the elevator, (the look is like some scenes in *Night of the Living Dead*), and then up to the second floor, and when our names are called out after we get up there, each of us is taken into a separate small area, curtained off into a room, where every word said in all the other curtained-off rooms comes to us in muffled, surreal, sci-fi tones.

And the physical setting itself has a kind of war movie feel too, primarily because of the temporary quality of the fabric walls—but more sober and reverent than *MASH*, it's more *So Proudly We Hail*. I'm told to undress, put my belongings in a plastic bag (a *plastic* bag! And why were the instructions so specific that we should wear "loose, comfortable" clothing, if we are to get rid of it all so quickly), and put on a hospital gown.

A very positive and chipper (chipper at 6:00 AM yet!) nurse, who manages too, at the same time, to be all business and to give the impression of considerable competence, hooks me up to an IV and our conversation is very casual (the weather, etc.), as though this is to be really no big event, thus heightening the surreal feel. There is a sort of pretense that I am not there to have a cancer in my kidney removed, that there are no life-death issues, that surgery like this is maybe what people usually do Thursday mornings; the word *cancer* is never mentioned—come to think of it, it never has been in my case. A friendly looking, compact man with facial hair and a very soft, benevolent manner comes in, introduces himself as the anesthesiologist (since my nephew became an anesthesiologist I am ready to love them all—and this guy looks so giving, thoughtful, and warm, I'll go along with anything he says; let me ask you, are there other qualities by which one can judge people in these circumstances?); and then he says, looking through some papers, in a tone that might be used to comment on the color of one's tie, "I see that you are having your left kidney removed this morning."

There is a needle in my arm by now (an IV is dripping into me for God knows what reason: they say it's a sedative, like we're in a Bette Davis movie, but why would I need a sedative? I'm not tense and if I am tense, so what? Isn't tension a reasonable response to the situation?), I'm wearing a little hospital robe open in the back I'm lying on a gurney, there is no way I can get off the gurney and run like hell, with anything like grace and manliness. Instead, I say, "No. The doctor wrote that only in order to reserve enough time in the O.R. just in case, but what is really going to happen is that he is only going to remove a tumor from my left kidney (quoting my surgeon! Here again identification with the oppressor) and please, I need to ask you to stop him if he looks like he is going to remove the kidney."

(On the subject of hospital gowns, surely there are designers who might have come up with something even more efficient, and less humiliating than these! and even if you have the dexterity to tie the top strings, the ones in back at your neck, surely there is no one in the world who might be able to tie the others for himself. It's like the strings are there because they want to make you feel responsible for your ass being exposed. But, while I'm on the subject, even worse, have you ever been forced into one of those paper ones? By opting for the paper, the administration doesn't have to worry about sending out laundry. You feel like a fool dressed in paper that slides everywhere, your dignity is out the door, but they save themselves the nuisance of sending out laundry!)

The response is a little laughter—not assurances, chuckles—like I'm joking with them! So in order to avoid being thought a paranoid nut, foolishly not trusting the word of my surgeon, and to avoid the awkwardness of getting off the gurney with my ass exposed and anything like dignity gone, I smile too. Then the anesthesiologist starts to talk to me about pain. He talks about subjectively rating my post-surgery pain on a scale of one to ten and offers me a choice of two pain-alleviating technologies. Before he finishes, the nurse intrudes, criticizing him for emphasizing and showing a preference for one over the other. I had been pleased with his emphasis, because I have no criteria from my experience to enable me to choose one over the other, but she is angry and Diana and I don't know where to look while the argument goes on (It's *So Proudly We Hail* now turning into *Mash!).* Soon things simmer down, I choose the morphine drip (I like the sound, the underworld feel, and he clearly prefers this method), he talks a little about pushing a button at six minute intervals (though I can't quite picture it, I nod my head and smile), we wait a while, Diana leaves and I'm wheeled away.

Next thing I know I'm in the recovery room and the surgeon is telling me that he had to remove the entire kidney. Here we go: worst-case scenario strikes and there's no way I can deal with it, it's after the fact! And he doesn't even seem apologetic. What happened to the *partial nephrectomy*, the *renal reconstruction*? At first I figure maybe I'm not hearing right! After all my caution, my clarity, and my insistence, he couldn't possibly have done that! The removal of a kidney is, to me, big stuff, but his comments are rather ho-hum. He points out again that the remaining kidney will take over the function of my now missing one. I now understand fully Ronald Reagan's experience in *Kings' Row* when he wakes up after surgery and realizes that his legs have been (needlessly) amputated.

In retrospect, the situation is worse than one might have believed. When I learn much later reading my file (an indulgence that has been guaranteed by the legislature in every state I've lived in) that the surgery was indeed done by a resident (though he does assure us in his write-up that the Master was in the OR throughout the surgery), I figure at first that the resident was not practiced in the surgery and made some error that left the removal of the kidney the only option, and a cover-up ensued. But, "The patient presented for a radical nephrectomy," it says and we know that I certainly did not. And nowhere in the write-up is there any suggestion that *removal of the tumor only* might have been part of the original plan. And logically that scenario of the beginner resident flubbing doesn't work, since the papers they gave me pre-op and the language used by the anesthesiologist indicate that the nephrectomy was the plan all along; there is no way I can understand these events except to think that, for whatever obscure reason, prior to the surgery I was lied to repeatedly about what was going to be done to my body! Ain't that a bitch! But in fact a system that is dishonest about who will be doing the actual cutting might be telling other lies too; that is, the difference between an honest response and a lie becomes for the practitioner unclear, muddy.

And my giving, thoughtful, warm, fuzzy anesthesiologist— where the hell was he when it became clear that the plan was to remove the kidney? Surely he heard me prior to surgery when I beseeched him not to allow a nephrectomy. Did he think I was kidding or did he dismiss me as a nut case? Or was it merely that, on the surgeon's turf, the surgeon knows best and brooks no questioning? Here's my fantasy: everyone is having a fun time in the OR, the anesthesiologist quotes me when he realizes what is about to happen to my kidney, and the surgeon and/or resident have quite a little chuckle about that. One would think that I took enough precautions, that I was clear enough—but unconscious in the O.R., I have no power and, of course, no say.

Since I have copies of the letter the surgeon wrote to Ernie describing his "intended" removal of the *tumor only* and of the write-up of the surgery itself in which the possibility of the removal of the *tumor only* is not even mentioned, one might wonder why I've not even contemplated suing. I'm not really sure why, but here are some suggestions. First, I'm not a suer; I have never engaged in any litigious behavior and it would feel odd to start now. Second, the kidney is gone and the consequences of that cannot be ameliorated; no matter what actions I take I cannot increase the number of kidneys I have. Third, were I to win a suit, the surgeon's malpractice insurance company loses money, he doesn't. I don't care about the fiscal situation of his insurance company; it's him I would want to punish. So much for the *frivolous* law suits we hear so much about!

(There is another, maybe even more cogent reason: I feel that I am essentially responsible for what happened. It's like with smoking: I could never sue a tobacco company, because I knew for at least the last twenty-five years of my smoking career that smoking had harmful physiological effects and I kept on smoking. I didn't even contemplate stopping before Sandra died. So, any problems that were engendered by smoking are my responsibility. In this present situation I had bad feelings repeatedly about what was taking place prior to surgery; yet I went ahead with it. I should have cancelled and put it off a few weeks, because I didn't like or understand the situation. Had I done that, had I listened to myself, things might have been different. So a big piece of the responsibility is mine.)

Then the surgeon tells me that he is about to take his son to Tahoe for a few days of skiing and that while he is away these few days, his associate will be around to see me in the hospital. So this is how he develops a surgery opening! Just cut out the kidney and skip town! Nobody mentioned to me before that he was not going be around. I don't like him, I won't miss him, but I resent his abandoning me to an unknown buddy of his, who will not, I am sure, be able to tell me anything I want to know, like why the kidney was removed and what the relationship is between its removal, the *radical nephrectomy* on the papers pre-op, and the initial comment by the anesthesiologist. In the recovery room; my mind is too blurry, things feel too murky, for me to raise any of this with him, all I want to do is go back to sleep, and I'm not even sure that I really heard it right and what will I do with the information anyway, weak, in bed, metal staples in me, tubes sticking out all over, and not quite aware nor thinking.

Some time later I'm aware of being pushed on a gurney off an elevator into a patient unit and that Diana, my daughters Annie and Ruthie, and my friend Paul are there waiting. It is at that point—it seems to me now, that it happens even before I get into the room—that a nurse introduces herself and welcomes me and begins immediately to ask me about my pain: how would I rank the pain on a scale of one to ten? I've done some reading myself and I know that this pain control is important, and the anesthesiologist made that clear too, but honestly, at this point I feel nothing except sleepy and awkward and very foggy, and she needs me to put figures on how much pain I have.

Because it seems so important to her, I am embarrassed to tell her that I don't have, or at least I don't have any awareness of any pain, which is to me the same as not having pain—I have very little awareness of anything—but I know she needs some numbers and without them I'll be here in the corridor all day, and frankly I need to get into bed fast and go to sleep. And I do want to please her, to do right by her; she will, after all be taking care of me for the next several days, so I want to stay on her good side. So I tell her *four* when I'm lying still, *seven* when I move at all, very proud that, in the mental shape I'm in at that moment, I've thought of breaking it down that way, but these numbers represent nothing except what I think she wants to hear and, in fact, she does seem relieved when I finally give them to her and she is able to tell me something that I interpret as orders to push the morphine button every six minutes. It's like those moments in movies when all movement, all action has stopped and the color has been bled out, until I give her numbers, and then, as soon as the numbers are out of my mouth, things begin moving again at a normal speed In wonderful Technicolor.

I'm nice, I'll do what she tells me to do, and I forget that what she told me to do is based on numbers I invented out of nothing in relation to my supposed experience of pain. Funny, once I start the regime I don't get any less foggy than I am at the moment, and it is true that nothing ever really hurts! Now for the first time in my life I'm a patient in hospital unit and will be there several days. Much of those days and nights are to be a haze, but I do remember, out of the incredibly surreal quality some feelings, some incidents and will try to describe them.

Every morning, very early, three young Asian men, in white jackets, come to see me. One of them, always in the middle and a little forward of the others, is able to express himself somewhat in English, the others say not a word and do not look to understand anything I say. Their primary interest seems to be around my ability to have a bowel movement, though they express interest too in whether or not I pass gas. These brief discussions about farting are for me the epitome of absurd—how can I take seriously questions about farting to begin with, let alone in English so heavily accented it is barely understandable. It's like an old Sid Caesar routine—and it's too bad that I'm not able to tape these early morning attempts at conversation; I am sure that the tapes would sell big.

I know that I am not allowed to eat or drink until I have a bowel movement, but none of them explains—at least I think none explains, since I have a great deal of trouble understanding even the middle one, the talker—how I am to have a bowel movement, having done enemas before surgery and having had nothing to eat since then. What is to have been digested? I'm not even sure what function these young men serve, what their role in the hospital hierarchy is: their English is not adequate to enable them to survive medical school, so they couldn't be medical students; perhaps interns or residents, but then shouldn't their interests be wider than bowel movements? I know that the middle one introduced himself to me, but I didn't get it. These visits are for me like a take-off on an absurdist ballet; they, my early morning ritual, are my *Trocadero Ballet*.

During my first two days (and nights), doing what I think the nurse has told me to do, I try compulsively to press the morphine button every six minutes. It's almost religious. Five-minute intervals would have been easier, especially with my being as groggy as I, not surprisingly, continue to be, the five-minute marks on the clock would surely help. But they said six, and I want to do what they said, so I spend a good deal of my time checking the clock, doing addition, and waiting to push. There is, of course, never a moment in which I am able actually to feel pain; the morphine obviates that. So there is no way I can check to see whether I really need the relief. They said six minutes, that one heals better without pain, and who am I to make a fuss, so every six minutes the button gets pushed.

There is a painting of anemones in my room, probably 20x24, and on the second night I find that it is not only anemones (I'd not noticed this before), but that there is also a wizard in the middle wearing formal clothes and a cape (he looks a lot like John Carradine, maybe in *Stagecoach*) and the petals of the anemones have become people engaged in unspeakable, mostly sadomasochistic, sexual acts, at the command of the wizard. People are getting hurt and there is blood everywhere in my room, dripping on the walls, on the floor—more blood than you might expect from their acts alone. I don't ask myself why there would be blood on the walls and floor—it is, after all, only a picture, even though it's animated—I question none of this. Somehow, the picture is hooked up with the clock, which does more than keep time; it enables, through some hidden mechanism, the dreadful changes that are constantly taking place in the painting! This activity in the strange, intriguing painting happens usually only when the door is closed, the lights are out, and there is no other sensory experience. I don't like it at all; I think that whatever committee chooses art for patient areas made a terrible, frightening mistake, a breach of taste. But there it is—especially at night.

The next day the anemones don't do much; there are people around all day and a certain amount of action. At night it starts again; but I notice too, in the dark, that the room is different, I know that I am in a different place, and that a woman is sitting at the door. I don't know how I've been transported, but I have a notion that the transfer was done by bus—like those vehicles in movies that transport prisoners to and from court—and the woman by the door is nobody I know. I realize that I have to call Diana before she leaves for the hospital in the morning to see me, so I call. It is 1:30 AM, but I know she'll understand the urgency; I need to get to her in time. I tell her that they have moved me and that there is a woman guarding the door and that she'd better call the nurses to find out where to go in the morning. She responds pleasantly, though sleepily, and a few minutes later a nurse comes to my room to ask how I am doing; the corridor light makes everything in the room clear, I tell her I am fine, ask her to leave the door open, and I realize finally that it is time to stop the morphine drip. And the subject of my morphine hallucinations is never broached by any of the staff.

Diana must have been sufficiently wigged out or concerned, not only about my delusions, but also about my poor judgment in calling her at so ungodly an hour, that she decides to spend the next night in my room on a "chair-bed" the nurse will get for her. I don't feel this at all necessary—I'd now spent many hours off morphine, but I am delighted that she will do it for me; it is not a physically comfortable situation (the *bed* part of chair-bed is a joke!), the sociology of hospitals does not allow much psychological comfort, and yet she's staying. It's an act of love. Late in the evening, we both go to sleep. I wake up at about 5:00 AM, feeling a little nausea, not a lot of nausea, but I'd been told to call the nurse if I'm at all uncomfortable. So I push the button for the nurse, hoping that I am not waking Diana. The nurse comes and Diana sleeps. I explain very quietly that I am feeling a little nausea, somewhat embarrassed because it really is just a very little.

She seems to take it in her stride and says that she will be right back with some medicine. She returns, injects the medicine into my IV tube—she says it's *droperidol*—and leaves. Almost immediately a wave of extreme cold travels down my body, beginning at my throat and spreading slowly down to my feet. I ring for the nurse and this time Diana wakes up because by now I have begun to have trouble breathing and the gasping makes loud noises!

The nurse does not come immediately. Diana runs to the nursing station (I'm really having trouble breathing) and a group comes running back with her . . . to watch me gasping and freezing. Blankets are thrown on me, but the gasping and icy feeling continue. Between gasps I manage to say that I need an antidote to the <u>droperidol</u> and people race out of the room and it seems to me that nothing is done for an eternity. A fourth year surgery fellow, a woman who'd introduced herself to me the day before as Natalie, saunters in, literally saunters; she is a large woman, over six feet tall, her long hair is rather unkempt, she looks like she just woke up (she probably did; it is, after all, the middle of the night) and she is wearing a medical school sweatshirt. She approaches me, puts a hand on my shoulder and asks, "Do you want to let go?"

I'm thinking that maybe the morphine has come back and that I am hallucinating again, but through my gasps I see Diana across the room staring in disbelief at this woman. I realize immediately that she must have been involved recently in a Death and Dying seminar and is proudly practicing what she thinks she was taught. Nonetheless I find myself yelling between gasps and through the shivering, "No. I need an antidote or something," instead of blowing her off with the fact that I had supervised Kubler-Ross during part of her psychiatric residency. And just at that moment, the nurse runs into the room, injects something into the IV tube, and as quickly as the attack came, it goes away and Natalie, by gum, has also slipped away. (Once in a while, these days, I think of this situation: I'm vulnerable, what if I had taken her seriously!) This event is never again mentioned by any personnel dealing with me; a situation in which I was afraid I was dying is apparently, after it's over, of little interest to anyone working there.

A physician comes to see me often; he introduces himself as the associate of my surgeon, but, just as I predicted, he is unable to explain the kidney removal, except to say that *they* couldn't get just the tumor out by itself. Nor does he ever comment on my drug reaction: he's a surgeon, not a drug person, so apparently it holds little interest for him. He is a youngish man, probably in his late thirties, big and burly—my image of him is smoking a cigar, but I know that that cannot be, indoors, in a hospital, in this state; it does however fit my general impression of him—and he is always followed by a train of younger people, obviously less informed about my situation than he, though it is never clear if they are medical students or residents. That it is the week before Christmas and that, having been admitted on a Thursday, much of my hospital stay is the week-end may excuse somewhat his attire: he wears something like what we used to call a *letter jacket*; it says *MGM Grand* on the front and *Boxing* on the back (I would not exactly call this appropriate) and it is hard not to relate his entrances with his entourage to those moments in boxing movies when the hero, in his robe, races down the hall toward the ring accompanied by trainers and lackeys. My three Asian regulars are sometimes, but only rarely, in his claque.

He asks few questions and his attitude indicates that it would not be quite appropriate for him to give me any information. Every time he comes to see me (I think it's daily), he is a bit jokey, but gruff, and never really funny. Of course, he might be giving his group oodles of essential information in the corridor before and after his visits with me, but nobody shares that with me. He too raises the issue of bowel movements (which seems to me actually a very private, indelicate matter to be talked about so publicly in front of a horde of white-jacketed kids), contributing to my concept of myself as a failure: not only have I been unamusingly delusional, but also here I am not getting on with very basic bodily functions. My belly is distended (a humiliating situation for me—I like to look good) and I am simply not able to will it away.

He tells me several times during my hospital stay that his associate, my surgeon, is expected back from skiing with his son any day now, but he never materializes. Strange, isn't it, that no one knows for sure when this man is to return; that neither the son nor he has a schedule, (if there is one, it is one to which I surely cannot be privy), that there are no plans, that no secretary knows when a boss is coming back. It's hard to believe, isn't it, that medical practices, hospitals, medical schools can operate that way, without schedules!

Attached to the index finger of my right hand is one of those clips that they explained to me measures the efficiency of my oxygen usage. Nursing personnel invariably fuss with it and with the machine it is attached to whenever they come into the room; they change the finger, flick the clip and the machine, and always seem unhappy with the reading, that is to gauge how well I am doing with oxygen. It is a ritual of theirs and I want to make them feel good by doing better by my oxygen, but apparently I can't do it. Since I am feeling pretty good and don't sense any real deprivation of oxygen, I suggest that perhaps the machine giving the reading—it actually looks pretty ratty—is not functioning properly. Generally they patronize me with a smile, until I finally prevail on someone to call the technician in charge of these machines and he comes to see what is going on. A charming, surprisingly understated, young Russian man, disheveled, but witty—he says, after looking things over, that he ought to change the machine and see what that might do. He leaves, comes back with a new machine, and surprise, surprise, my oxygen usage is exemplary!

I am scarcely aware of other patients on the floor. I have contact with all kinds of employees, and, it may be because of the proximity to Christmas, I see almost no other patients. There is, however, a couple, both looking to be in their late fifties, that passes my room at least once daily, he wearing a robe, dragging an IV pole, she, apparently his wife, visiting him. They look right, like we could be friends. We nod at each other as they pass. Gradually the nods last longer, and, although few if any words are articulated, it's as though we begin to know each other.

One day they are carrying a small dog; Diana, who can never let a dog just pass by, goes to them and after making nice with the dog learns that from time to time the wife sneaks the dog into the hospital because seeing and playing with his dog delights the husband. Mutual introductions occur. Several days later, they stop by my room to say that he is being discharged that day. We chat a bit and learn that they live just a few blocks from us and that he is an academic, an economist. Clearly we have new friends in the neighborhood! We exchange phone numbers and there are mutual assurances that we will contact each other. We congratulate him on leaving the hospital, but his wife hesitantly says that actually the news is not that good, that he is being discharged because there is nothing more that can be done for his liver cancer. Holy shit! There goes a budding friendship! I am humiliated by the fact that I simply don't have the energy to become involved with a couple where mourning is likely to be what the situation will call for soon. We are not able ever to get it together to call them, and she never calls us.

Visitors. I certainly have phone calls, and flowers, and visitors. I like having Diana around and Annie too, although with Annie I have to communicate and that is too much like work, so I take a deep breath and ask that she not come so often. Ruthie has gone with her husband for a Christmas trip to visit her in-laws in Cleveland, so I am spared (as is she) having to ask her not to come so often.

During the high point of my morphine experience, my close friend Paul comes in with his wife; I don't recognize them, I ask them who they are, and am a little suspicious that they are lying when they tell me. Other friends drop by when I am my old rational self and happily all know to stay only a very short time; I guess they pick up that I don't have the energy for conversation. The last time I saw Charlie before I went into the hospital, he commented that he will drop by to see me, since he's frequently in the building. He never shows and I am disappointed. Though he never said he'd come by, I am disappointed too that Richard Caplin never shows up. I certainly have nothing to say to anybody and it is a drain on me when people do show up and yet it bothers me that these two men don't come by. I don't know what exactly I want from them, but it sure seems that I do want something; maybe it's because they are the only two guys that I trust in this medical arena. I have lots of phone calls from friends and family everywhere and since they can't see me, I am able to do my usual number of "Everything is terrific."

After a few days, I am allowed to go beyond ice chips and start a liquid diet, which includes *Jello* and later, a variety of puddings, generally a sickly beige, the color alone signaling inedibility. I notice that no matter where I am—in bed, on a chair—whoever brings my tray of unattractive, unappealing, to me almost inedible food is always able to find a place to leave it, not too far from me, and yet strangely inaccessible. I simply can never get the tray to me. I just can't compete with their expertise at inaccessible tray placement: I have an IV, I have a catheter, I have staples across half my belly, so I can't move around with much agility. At every mealtime, then, I have to call someone to move the tray so that I can get at it, in order then to be able to reject it as food. The original tray bringers are very efficient at leaving the room before I can ask them to move the tray.

One blessing though is that the nurses, clearly out of sympathy with my dietary problems, think to bring me raspberry tea Snapple, my very first, and it is a life-changing experience. Another is that Annie discovers great ice cream in the visitor's dining room and brings me as much as I am willing to eat. I exist happily, then, on a diet of Snapple and ice cream, though not together. This situation, that is, food service in the hospital, brings to mind the time that my daughter Ruthie, age seven or eight, was in the hospital for a couple of days to watch a very sore ankle (it turned out to be nothing). One of those days, during a moment when we were not around, she was asked to fill out a form to select her meals for the next day. She did what she was asked, of course there was no supervision, and the following day at each meal she got several containers of salad dressing (no salad), butter (no bread), and a few vegetables here and there. No one on the unit went over her selections, and no one in the kitchen found it a problem to be sending out so strange an array to a pediatrics unit.

A woman, who bathed me one day, comes into my room the following day and tells me that today I will wash myself. The day before she sponge-bathed me and, when she was finished, handed me the washcloth, turned around and told me to wash my *privates* (her word, uttered in a Spanish accent, making it difficult to understand at first—and my *privates* have been pretty public so far in the hospital); I did (though I must say that the presence of a catheter adds a freaky dimension and complicates the procedure some and at this point all thoughts of modesty are out the window) and felt that this was a reasonable division of labor. This time, she pushes my big old armchair (by no means a wheel chair—it's a heavy armchair and, in addition, I'm in it) to the sink, hands me soap and washcloth, and leaves. I still have a catheter and IV (complicating the pushing for her) and that plus my staples make the washing virtually out of the question for me, or at least a skill I will master only with instruction and a lot of practice. I can't move much, I feel terribly woozy (more about that later), I'm sitting there in front of the mirror, and I'm having trouble arranging myself physically to begin. I can turn the faucet on, that's about it; then I need to rest. Showers are how I bathe, anyway, and here I'm supposed to do something, seated opposite a sink faucet, essentially immobile, and with no instruction!

Nurses keep urging me to walk, schlepping the IV pole, the bag into which the catheter empties, and whatever other paraphernalia is attached to me. It is a logistic nightmare, but that isn't the half of it. Diana accompanies me and supports me, because I feel so precarious and unbalanced, and the possibility of falling, with all these attachments, looms large. Very quickly, in addition to all these problems, after just a few steps, I am dizzy and terribly out of breath, and, although I think that that must be the natural consequence of my surgery (so I don't bother the nurses with that information), it shortens the length and number of my walks. The nurses do see, however, that I am sometimes up and about, and seem very happy with

57

me. It's like in Dr. Kildare movies, when Lionel Barrymore, Dr. Gillespie, tells the kid that he can walk, that he can do it, and the pleasure that he (Barrymore) gets when the kid takes a few steps.

Throughout the hospitalization, I remain on hydroxyurea for the leukemia. When the nurses come to give me those pills, they put on rubber gloves for the transaction—they don't do it for any of the other drugs they give me. I'm taking a drug that nurses need to protect themselves from! No one says a word; they just put the gloves on and hand me the paper cup with the pills; the pills go directly from cup to my hand, their hands contact only the paper of the cup, a barrier to the pills, and yet, the gloves! Shouldn't there be a conversation now about toxicity and why it's OK for me? Do they think I don't notice the gloves? If they need to protect themselves from my drug, my God! what is this drug going to be doing to me?

I do have a gripe with a particular linguistic fancy commonly used by much of the nursing personnel that deals with me. The addition of the words *for me* to a request is a strange usage indeed; when they want me, for example, to take a pill, they often say, "Swallow this pill *for me*." First time I hear it, my grogginess and general discomfort preclude my asking, "Why should I swallow anything for you? Swallow it yourself." Later, because I hear it so often, I become sufficiently inured to it, that it just sweeps by me. Now, in retrospect, I wonder how the concept arose and how they allow themselves to communicate anything so infantilizing to adults. It's even a few rungs below the almost universal freedom among hospital personnel (interestingly, except for doctors who address me as *Mister* or *Doctor*) to call me by my first name.

And then there is that shade of green that exists, I think, nowhere but on hospital walls. You know the color. How did it come about? The mixture could not have happened as a way to make patients comfortable—it doesn't! Soothing? Well, it doesn't soothe me! An esthetic choice? No way! It can't be. Somebody mixed it once and other people all over this country have chosen it. I don't think that the choice is forced, so why do they pick it? Paint stores have what seem like an infinite number of colors. Maybe it's supposed to match scrubs. But even scrubs seem to have changed to blue.

During the six days of this hospitalization I am unable to learn how to operate the TV, literally just a few inches from the side of my face. I've watched TV in many places—the history of TV, after all, took place during my life, but this one works apparently like none I've ever dealt with. I don't feel like watching TV and anyway, in order to see the screen, my body or at least my head, has to be turned to one side, a position I cannot sustain for long; but that is certainly not the point—it is there supposedly for my use and I can't figure out how to use it. Nurses show me, but I can't replicate what they do and it's embarrassing to keep asking; and even when they do it for me, the quality of TV reception is like 1949.

Oh, and the bed! Since it's cranked up so that I'm supposed to be able to sit up during the day, as time passes, even though the mattress is raised a bit at the knees, I gradually slide down so that most of me, much of the day, is scrunched up in the bottom of the V that the bed makes. I am afraid to push myself back up, because it feels like the exertion will rip apart my incision. I think that what is responsible for the slide is the slippery thing under the sheet that is supposed to protect the mattress from me—but no one will remove it, even when the catheter precludes my wetting the bed. There is nothing to protect me from it and I keep sliding.

When the day of my discharge arrives, I am told that as soon as the staples are removed (I didn't even know that they had stopped using stitches!), I'll be leaving. Nobody, however, comes to remove them. I know that I have to be out of there: it's getting closer to Christmas day, so many beds are empty and it seems that most of the personnel is beginning to be away on vacation. In addition, this place is quite obviously psychopathogenic, i.e. it is crazy making. So, at any rate, after five days I want out, and I keep asking the nurses when the person will come to remove the staples. Finally, he is there, my expert staple remover: a medical student! I am sure that he has had as little experience doing this as, say, Diana, who's been sitting there with me now for hours awaiting this arrival; we could somehow have done this together and been out of there hours before!

Instead of complaining, I expose the area, seeing for the first time the incision from just above my navel across my abdomen and around to the side (remember that I'd asked for a small one? What if I hadn't mentioned size?), and actual metal staples! But I take comfort in his reply to my question that it won't hurt. I actually relax, but when he pulls the first one out I realize that either he lied when he said it wouldn't hurt or he doesn't know (I promise you that he will know when asked in the future), because the pain is sharp and terrible and I feel that I've jumped to the ceiling. And it doesn't get any better. The removal of each staple shocks me with the pain and there are many to remove. And finally the procedure is over and, as promised, I can leave the hospital.

I do indeed survive the procedure, reinforced in my not so new view of the medical establishment: these people lie, they are not rational, they often don't know what they are talking about, one cannot trust them—your life is in their hands and you cannot trust them, the left hand doesn't know what the right is doing, the patient's judgment and intelligence are certainly not to be taken into account, it is rarely the patient and his/her comfort that is of major concern, it is the procedure (no matter who does it!) that needs to be accommodated, medical students cannot be blamed for what they are ordered to do, irony is an important ingredient in what happens in hospitals and the staff has been trained never to be cognizant of irony, and, most important one needs oneself to be (or at least to feel that one is) in charge of one's medical treatment.

Diana drives us home.

IV

*In which, after my discharge from the hospital, I try
a number of approaches to my medical condition
and the problems that that condition causes, none
of which approaches makes me feel any better.*

When we get home, my delight at being out of the hospital turns very quickly into anxiety about and disappointment with how dizzy and lousy I feel and how much effort it takes just to get out of the car, to walk up the ten stairs, and to get into the house. I am panting, gasping, and through the gasps I hear my fast and horrendously loud heartbeat as I walk very slowly and precariously down the hallway to our bedroom. I'm afraid I'm not going to make it! I can unzip my fly, but that's as far as I can go in dealing with my clothing; I sit on the edge and Diana brings my legs up onto the bed to join the rest of me. It's a terrible feeling, unlike anything I've ever experienced; very candidly, although I would certainly not tell anybody, it feels like I'm about to die. I don't want to add panic to my problems right then, so I rationalize the feeling. Being a novice, I am able to convince myself that everyone fresh out of the hospital, five days after serious surgery like a nephrectomy, is going to be unable to walk five feet without feeling completely winded and needing to sit down. Comfort in numbers allays the panic.

As the days go by, having rejected Diana's offer to help me do it ("there's nothing wrong with me, I can handle this perfectly well myself!"), I shower seated on a plastic chair, panting much of the time and feeling that, unless I am very vigilant, I will keel over any moment; I thus shower very slowly and that causes Diana to pop in every so often, a pop-in that I resent, since it means that she too is worried about me there and, if she is worried, then the possibilities are real and—well, by now you know my proclivities.

An upstairs neighbor once told me at a condominium meeting that one ought to engage supermarket checkers in small talk while they ring things up, because it's important to affirm their humanity (I felt that there was something condescending in his notion that without his chit-chat, their "humanity" dissipates—but *live and let live* is my credo!) He is known to be "handy" around the house, that is, he is comfortable with tools and knows how to fix things. Even though we are not close friends, because she is feeling desperate for my safety, Diana asks him if he would put up grip bars for us in the shower; we have already bought them and they are on hand. He says that he has to think about it and then three days later he stops her outside to say that because of issues of liability he thinks it best not to do it. What's supposed to happen with my "humanity"? Maybe "humanity" becomes an issue only when one's name is known only from a nametag! Maybe physical proximity decreases his wish to affirm! Well, at least it took him three days to get up the nerve to tell us. You might have guessed that this transaction does not bring us closer. So we ask a plumber who comes to our house to fix something else to do it and so far no problems with liability.

After a bit of time in bed, mostly watching great old movies (I'd prepared a list before I went into the hospital and Diana was able to get the videos for me—isn't she something!)—I can't concentrate well enough to read, I begin to come close to accepting this situation, although it is frightening and I have not expected it. Actually I do not expect anything, because, before I left the hospital, no one talked to me about anything in relation to my surgery and about what to expect later. One nurse did share with me the name of an over-the-counter antacid that did very well both for her and her husband. (It has apparently not yet been put together that the hiatal hernia that showed up on the CT Scan and my heartburn might be related or, if it has, no one has yet told me anything—that may be the rubric of another specialty). Over the next few days the breathlessness and fatigue lessen some (especially when I am in bed, not doing anything), but do not entirely go away. I figure that in a matter of weeks, if I make it that long, I will be back to normal and with that in mind, a week after leaving the hospital, we set off to see the surgeon for the appointed post-op visit.

Seated in the office are the surgeon and the middle Asian fellow, still in his very white jacket (it's not a white coat, it's a jacket; the difference seems to be hierarchical, but who knows). After the obligatory exchange of niceties, the surgeon tells me that the surgery has been very successful, that while composed of malignant cells, the tumor had margins (margins?), lymph nodes reveal no cancer cells, there seems to be no reason to worry about a recurrence, that from his point of view, everything is hunky-dory.

I ask him why, given what he's saying about the tumor, the entire kidney had to be removed. "Well," he says, "we had to. There was no way we could get the tumor out by itself." No further explanation, no details, no diagrams. This is the man, whose artistry, I've been told, is such that he is able to take a kidney out onto a table and work on it meticulously to remove a tumor and then put the kidney back nicely where it belongs! Clearly he knows tumors better than I, he's seen it, he is the big maven—and yet I cannot altogether let go of my idea that he has removed my kidney in order to save time so that he can leave at a good hour to take his son skiing (my thinking being that it's more work and time to carve a tumor out of something than simply to schlep out the whole kidney). Well, I have to live with that possibility, since no one offers me any more coherent explanation of the number of things that seem so suspicious.

Quite a while later, I learn that immediately after the surgery, he speaks to Diana who is in the relatives' area waiting to hear about the outcome of the surgery. He tells her that he removed the entire kidney in order to eliminate the possibility of the cancer spreading. This is not the reason he's given me and it is a bit lame: he's commented on the margins (i.e., the tumor was encapsulated, no extra little bits leeching off the whole), he noted that lymph nodes showed no involvement. So what is he talking about and why would he not have told me this prior to the surgery? If the goddamn thing is going to metastasize, those nasty little cells would very well already be moving up my blood stream to other organs, so removing the kidney is not likely to impede the progress of the cancer. And again, without being asked, he does assure her, as he has me, that the right kidney will soon take over the function of the left and do the work of both.

He then has me unbutton my shirt in order to check out my eleven inch, red, angry-looking scar, about which he says only very favorable, admiring things. (Well, what else can he say! He made the goddamn thing!) When I comment on its size and redness and general obviousness, he says that as time goes by it will recede and be barely evident. (Now, years later, while it has ceased being red, in other ways what he said has not quite happened; but Diana does say that it is not as obvious as it seems to me.) I can't quite share his delight and I am completely floored when he says that there is no reason to see him again, that my primary physician, Richard, can follow me now for whatever needs to be done. ("What needs to be done to follow up?" "Well, that's something you and your doctor will be able to work out together.")

This man has removed my kidney, I am gasping for breath, I continue to sit on a chair to shower, I am scarred in what is to me a most disfiguring, revolting way, I am frightened despite his glib reassurance that the cancer will not recur—and even if it doesn't recur, I don't have any longer a safety net if anything at all goes wrong with my one kidney—and here he is, blowing me off. First he doesn't see me in the hospital and now the whole thing is over for him. Rejected by a suitor I never really cared for! And it's a terrible blow. I hate feeling scorned! There is, however, not much I can do about any of that, so we say goodbye and leave. But I am perplexed and disturbed and very unhappy. Let me mention here that we, Richard Caplin and I, decide later that the follow-up will be annual CT scans for five years, even though my having only one kidney precludes the use of contrast, thus rendering the scan at best murky.

Trust me when I tell you that I'm having a terrible time. Just one example: one day the universal remote I use stops relating to cable for the TV. I call the phone number for service etched on the remote and speak to a very engaging woman, who promises help. She wants to know the serial number on the cable box. That means that I have to get up from the couch, walk the six or seven feet to the TV, lift the box and read her the number on the bottom. By the time I've tilted the box in order to read the number, I am gasping and so out of breath that I cannot speak. The solution, of course is to sit down—she will wait, of course, but as soon as I sit, I realize that in that position the serial number is no longer available to me and I simply cannot stand again to get it or to get a pencil so I can write it down once I get back up to it and I am too out of breath to explain the situation to her. So, desperate and gasping, I manage to call out to Diana who is in another room, she comes flying in, ready for any emergency, and I beseech her to take over the call. Finally cable is restored!

When I get out of bed or even out of a chair, if I stand right up, I am very dizzy and the breathlessness is terrible and frightening. So I learn automatically to sit up on the side of the bed (or the edge of the chair) a while, before standing. I have to give up my normal bouncing out of bed, singing, for a more contemplative mode where I search for something for my mind to do, while I sit there just waiting for a little time to pass. And it works, and that pleases me enormously, not only because I avoid that terrible feeling, but also because I feel finally that I can be in control of something.

I keep my bi-weekly appointments with Charlie (remember? my leukemia man) and when I comment about how the smallest effort very quickly causes me shortness of breath, he suggests that perhaps it has to do with the surgery, that maybe a small clot ended up in my lungs; he has his office set up a new appointment with the surgeon who, two weeks prior, had as much as said that he never wanted to see me again. We return to see him.

When we get to his office, Diana, Annie (remember? my older daughter), and I, the receptionist is so concerned about my breathlessness that, as she has me sit down, asks me questions about my heart, indicating her concern that I am in heart failure. Well, I'm not, the gasping does stop when I sit, and we soon are called into the surgeon's office. He examines me a little—he even has a stethoscope!—says that my heart and lungs sound fine, but to assure ourselves that there is no lung problem as a result of the surgery, he immediately schedules by phone a lung scan for forty five minutes from then. The lung scan is to be done in a building across the street, for me a huge distance to walk. We walk, rather we trek, very slowly, stopping now and then, lots of support, physical and moral, from Diana and Annie.

We arrive at the place where lung scans are done about fifteen minutes prior to the appointment time, but that seems little excuse for the fact that no one comes to the window to find out who we are. We notice the wall signs that indicate that we are next to the psychiatric services, like coming home for me. We wait, we call out to the people we see inside the reception area, and finally someone responds, takes the required information, and tells us to be seated. The setting is a t-shaped situation, the corridor we've come on is the long leg, and the office is just to the right, where our corridor ends, on a shorter leg (psychiatry is to the left). The waiting area, not visible from the office (because it's on the long part of the T), is a small room off the main corridor, with a windowed wall separating it from the corridor. The large upholstered furniture and the coke and candy machines make the room seem rather askew and considerably smaller and tighter than reasonable, but the rather toney English magazines are a cut above what we're used to.

I am feeling terrible, sleepy, out of breath, with waves of nausea, and we remain seated, unattended to, and, of course, unseen for longer than any of us expected. Twice one of us (not me) goes up to the window to remind them that we are there and we are told that as soon as the technician gets back from the in-patient unit we will begin, that in-patient requests take precedence over out-patient ones (this makes no sense to me—in-patients are there all day and night, out-patients have schedules, they need to make a trip to the hospital and then go back to whatever they have to do; and furthermore they did give me an appointment just an hour or so ago; they should have known what was going on with their schedule), and that we should be seated, it won't be long.

After a wait of more than an hour past the scheduled appointment time, that is it's now 5:40 PM (what kind of working hours do these people have?), the elevator doors open, a woman wheeling a very large piece of equipment gets off and passes us on her way into the office—I'm afraid there is a Lucille Ball quality here. Some time later she comes back and tells us that it had taken her a very long time to get an elevator, that elevators are a big problem in the medical center, and she goes on about the problems that an employee pushing equipment has to deal with in this setting. Feeling that one more phrase from her will cause me to pass out from fatigue, breathlessness, anger—take your pick—I interrupt to say, as kindly as my mood and physical state allow, "Look, please, I'm not at all interested in your work problems, I only need to get this lung scan done."

She responds that she is just trying to explain why we'd had to wait. I say, mustering all the energy I can from the very scant pool that remains, that I don't need an explanation, that I'm not interested in why we had to wait, that we'd had an appointment for a particular time and that that's when we should have been seen. She responds that it is people like me who make everything difficult for people who are simply doing their job. Although I notice that Diana and Annie have that look on their face telling me that they need to be far away from this conversation and are hoping that I will not respond, and wishing that they might fly away from the area, because they fear that something terribly caustic will emerge from my mouth, I say only, "You are blaming the victim." She responds, "See. There you go, putting yourself in the role of victim."

I don't have the strength or energy to stand up and kill her. Instead I say very quietly, trying to express as little anger as I can, "Please. This conversation is over. Let's get the scan done." She goes away, another woman, very pleasant, verbal, and articulate, comes over, takes me in to do the scan.

Here's what happens. I sit in a chair with my head near a contraption so that I'm breathing some kind of mist sprayed every so often over about a five minute period. What I'm breathing is radioactive (I can't quite believe I'm putting my self in this position; I don't like radiation, no one I know likes radiation, we marched in the fifties against radiation!) and some device is recording how this radioactive material distributes itself in my lungs. Then I lie on a table in a variety of positions so my lungs can be seen from lots of angles, i.e., the lungs are being checked out essentially in 3-D, and . . . I pass the test. My lungs are fine. But the lingering question is that if this very nice woman is available to do the scan at this point, why didn't she do it to begin with, when we got there? I suppose it is possible that there is only one piece of equipment, but that wouldn't justify the number of employees sitting around, now would it?

A week later, on my birthday, the shortness of breath gets so bad that I feel I have to go in to see Charlie without an appointment, and, of course, it turns out that he isn't in that day. So they have me see a nurse practitioner, who is the first person to tell me that erythropoietin, secreted by the kidneys, is involved in spurring the formation of red cells and that, if I have only one kidney, it's possible that it's not making enough erythropoietin to keep my hemoglobin and hematocrit where they should be. Keep in mind the reassurance I'd been given about the remaining kidney taking over for the one removed! In the meantime, after conferring with other people, she thinks it would be wise for me to go off the hydroxyurea for five days and then go back on half the amount I've been on. (I must confess here that I extend my abstinence from hydroxyurea an additional five days, I suppose just in order to feel that I am somewhat in control of what is happening to me.

I mention to her, as an aside, that almost every time I swallow food, I have a terrible burning pain high up in my chest. She explains about the hiatal hernia (Wow! There is an occasional person who is willing to check stuff out from my file!) and gives me a prescription for Prilosec, something that will prevent the pain. (Here's how it stops the pain. The lining of the stomach has a large number of microscopic pumps that pump acid into the stomach to aid in the digestion of food. If a person has a hiatal hernia, though, some of the acid pumped into the stomach leaks up to the esophagus and boy, that can really hurt! This is the acid reflux we hear so much about these days. Prilosec inhibits some of the acid pumps in the stomach, so that what leaks into the esophagus is appreciably less acidic and, therefore, causes no pain.)

Oh, happy, happy birthday! I do what she says and after a few days I feel almost normal again. And no more pain when I eat! And the relief continues. Charlie comes back and we continue on this half-as-much routine, I feel almost good, and my white count, though a little high is stable. But I'm not getting rid of the disease and that means that, in the not too distant future, things will go haywire and I will die, a thought which, after all this agony, is, of course, frequently on my mind.

And so we go on. We are in a routine. And then, after five or six more months of status quo—from my point of view, five or six months closer to death—Charlie, as he had indicated initially, is ready to put me on Interferon. The major point of Interferon is that it's supposed to enhance body immunity and it has also been shown to inhibit cell growth—a dandy combination for certain kinds of cancers. Generally, when a person feels a little sick and fluey, and, here I am simplifying considerably, that feeling comes about because the natural Interferon in the body is mobilizing to help the immune system deal more efficiently with whatever the source of the infection is; that is to say, using, mobilizing Interferon causes that fluey feeling—at the same time that it (the Interferon) is doing you good. This then is the source of the warning that Interferon might make one feel like he/she has a little flu.

First a nurse teaches me how to inject myself subcutaneously and I feel very good about that, because first, it's always nice to learn a new skill and also, it seems to me that a drug with Interferon's rep, combined with injection instead of oral ingestion, makes for great power against any disease and very likely I'll be on safe ground in no time. She demonstrates two places to inject: in my thigh and in my belly; I find the belly possibility so loathsome, so revolting that I stick (a pun, alas!) exclusively to my thighs. I am warned about side effects ("it might feel like you've got a little flu"), but I know for sure, especially after the first week of working up to nine million units (when you're dealing with millions, you know this is serious stuff, so I am able to assure myself again that this is certain to do the trick), with no side effects (I am sure that since there are no side effects at the beginning when the stuff is new to my system, it will be easy sailing), that I will be OK.

Well, I am, unfortunately, very, very wrong; it doesn't work out that way at all. After a few weeks, in addition to the nuisance and upset and embarrassment of frequent vomiting (the embarrassment for me is especially great when I'm in someone else's living room), there is the fact that when I wake up in the morning or from one of the two naps that I now need every day, my first thought is, "When can I go back to sleep." I always feel at least somewhat sick to my stomach. There is so much of my hair on the bathroom floor each morning that sweeping becomes my new compulsion; and what hair remains on my head is straighter and finer than it has ever been. In addition, I taste salt all the time, even when I'm not eating, even when I'm eating ice cream—a very annoying turn of events, one that nobody has mentioned to me. And I just never feel right.

I do enjoy the romance of self-injection, and Diana and I manage still to be able even to travel, obsessed (and maybe even titillated) though I am about what the hotel maids will think is going on with all those syringes in wastebaskets and needing to schedule everything so that I can sleep some during the day. There are some inconveniences to my routine, of course, but I'm not going to take any of this assault lying down (again, a joke, in case you missed it); I will not be put off from doing the things that make my life my life. Whatever the inconvenience, whatever the struggle, I have to keep living the life I own and I cannot allow myself to acquiesce to the temptations that the sickness and/or the drugs bring.

One evening, my friend Gloria calls to tell me that a friend of hers, very sick with what I remember as non-Hodgkin's Lymphoma, in addition to making use of high-level Western medicine, had seen a Chinese practitioner in the city and he'd felt that the Chinese medical intervention had been very helpful, that she (the Chinese doctor) was very gifted and amazingly helpful to him. "Well, what the hell," I think, "a whole civilization has been able to thrive on it, maybe there's something to it, Gloria is very smart and her friend is likely not stupid and knows what has affected him, and anyway, what harm can it do." My daughter Ruthie, always spiritual and about to become a good Buddhist, is delighted with the possibilities and with what she certainly sees as my new flexibility. I clear it with Charlie who does not quite laugh at me and we make an appointment to see this much-lauded woman.

I get there a few minutes before the appointed time and open the door to the suite. There is a short hallway with a couple of clinical type rooms on either side and a couple straight ahead. There seems to be no waiting area. But tacked to a bulletin board in the hallway is a letter, extravagantly lauding the work this doctor had done with him, signed by Stan Getz. I wait a while standing in the hallway (that the Stan Getz letter is there for me to read indicates to me that I am supposed to wait there, standing) and soon the doctor comes out, her earlier patient leaves, and she brings me to another room in her warren. She is a very ordinary looking middle class Asian woman with a very pronounced Asian accent. I am embarrassed to tell you that it is difficult to understand anything she says to me. I need to ask her to repeat almost everything she says, but I am not willing to let anything go by not understood.

I tell her that I've read Getz's letter with considerable interest, she smiles, and I, wise-ass me, am unable to refrain from saying, with what I ambivalently think of as exquisite timing, "But, you know, he died soon after he wrote you." She nods and, apparently not to be outdone, quick as a bunny, says, "That was because he didn't do what I told him. He was having sex with young girls." Countless questions arise in my mind: How did she happen to counsel him in this area? Was it because the girls were young or just that he was having sex? Does having sex with young girls deplete one of chi more than sex with people one's own age? How did she learn that he had disobeyed? Etc. It would have been awkward to ask about any of this—there are issues of privacy and, more important, a man, a great saxophone player and innovator, after all, is dead—so, of course, I still wonder. But I decide that, after this crazy attempt of mine at *gotcha* about Getz, I am going to be taking this, my Eastern incursion, seriously and will give it all the chance I can.

There is a framed motto hanging above the door in the office to the effect that when God closes doors for us, He opens windows; a very nice thought, I suppose, but with only strained relevance to my current situation. If I really get into it, I suppose, it might be that if Interferon (the door) proves not to be useful, Chinese medicine is the window that opens up.

The doctor interviews me, disapproves of my taking Interferon (as though it's something I'm having a lot of fun with—though different from sex with young girls), has me practice some Chi Q'ong exercises, which she tells me I must do for an hour every day, does some very painful acupuncture, mostly in my legs, says she is calling in a prescription for Chinese herbs, gives me directions how to cook them up and drink the tea, instructs me to eat young female chicken, never male, (maybe Getz misunderstood this part: young female chickens→young chicks→young girls), tells me specifically which herb store in Chinatown to go to, gives me an appointment for one week hence, and tells me, in response to my questioning her about Medicare payments and Blue Cross that I ought to check with Blue Cross to see if her services are covered (they are not) and that her fee is $200 a visit. And then Diana and I are off to Chinatown, a few blocks away.

As everyone might suppose, here as in any big city, there is no place to park in Chinatown. So the plan is that Diana drives, parks in a no-parking zone where I sit at the wheel while she is in the herb store. She runs over and in the few minutes she is gone, I have to move the car a few times to make room for delivery trucks. My anxiety level is rising! And then she is out; but her arms are empty. She says that it will take them ten or fifteen minutes to weigh the herbs and get them together and during that time how would I like her to get us a barbecued duck (should the duck be female too?) in the store down the block? I like the idea very much, she goes off, gets the duck, then comes back with the herbs, and drives us home. The herbs cost about $70 for a week's supply (the duck is $7). The fact that this is getting a little costly assures me that it is going to work; you get what you pay for, right?

Once home, I begin cooking up the tea. I follow her directions compulsively: toiling and troubling, fire burning, cauldron bubbling. And there it is: the tea, the liquid product, is vile—the odor, the look, everything about it is vile, with an eye-of-newt quality, and yet I am sure that it will be all right to drink. Here too I am wrong. The drinking experience is terrible, it is foul, it is unbearable. Everything about me is so tentative and drinking something so awful starts me vomiting and, when that is over, since I committed myself, I feel I have to return to finish the tea, the fear of retching always on my mind. The duck, a bit later in the day, is different: it is not only delicious, but there are three legs!

Over the week I practice the breathing exercises an hour a day and the urge to vomit from the loathsome herb tea lessens some, but never goes away, and there is no way to predict when the retching might begin. On my return visit a week later, I explain that drinking the tea is a terrible and nauseating experience and she says that she will change the prescription and, without sacrificing its potency, make the tea more drinkable. (If she can change it now to be tolerable, why did I have to put up with it so vile for a week?) I ask if we can get the herbs elsewhere in the city where parking is less problematic and she says that we can't. No explanation. With what seems like hundreds of Chinese herb stores in this city, why only this one? A cousin, perhaps? I suggest that a weekly fee of $200 is somewhat beyond what we expected and she responds that I can be seen every other week.

We then do, she and I, what we had done the week before—breathing and acupuncture. When we pick up the herbs, this time two weeks worth, the cost is $120; since the first week was $70, I'd expected the price to be $140. I don't know if the herb guy is discounting on a double purchase or charging arbitrarily; I suspect the latter, but there are no clues, no prices listed. We continue the routine for another couple of months, but when I notice that my white count is consistently going up instead of down and, even though I acknowledge that she may be right, that it may be a result of the Interferon, I am reluctant to give the Interferon up, since it is probably the only chance that Western medicine affords me. I am beginning to think more seriously and suspiciously about the relevance of Stan Getz and his letter, why it is posted, and her comments about it.

I decide finally, despite my reluctance to hurt the doctor's feelings, to terminate my involvement with Chinese medicine. True, I rarely vomit from the tea now and I kind of like the breathing stuff (the acupuncture though remains always, for me, unpleasant and painful), but the whole thing is very inconvenient and, more to the point, I'm getting worse. And I've got to give me credit—I did try! It's all very disappointing: I'd committed myself to it, I wanted it to work, did everything wholeheartedly that I was supposed to do, and, my ambivalence notwithstanding, I liked the possibility that a joint East-West approach was going to do it. So now I am back to a wholly Western approach.

We manage, then, to get through the next four or five months (again four or five months even closer to death), but my white count is still higher than it should be and, of course, bone marrow aspirations reveal the presence still of the Philadelphia chromosome. So Charlie adds ara-C to my daily routine. Ara-C is one of the older chemotherapy drugs, which has been around and in use for many decades. It's been shown to be useful in acute and chronic leukemias and lymphomas.

Every evening, then, I take two syringes—one with Interferon, the other with ara-C and inject one in each thigh. I come to be highly skilled and get much satisfaction from the ritual: the alcohol swabs to each thigh, the preparation of the syringes, the little push on the plunger creating the arc of interferon or ara-C shooting into the air, then the injections themselves, followed by some more alcohol swabbing. I do like the ritual, but the side effects increase and the white count and Philadelphia chromosome don't budge.

I feel a little sorry for Charlie who seems frustrated that his attempts only increase side effects; I can see that he is trying hard and feels bad. I am personally very disappointed when he finally says after a couple of months that the combination of Interferon and ara-C is not being effective and that we will go back to Hydroxyurea. I am terribly concerned that the combination has not worked, but relieved that I won't be suffering those damned side effects. I am going to die in a minute, but I won't have those side effects. The hydroxyurea at least brought my white count down to normal; but I know, alas, that this drug will have no effect on the basic disease, nor can it increase my life expectancy. There is little I can do, but I simply cannot acquiesce to the likelihood of never reaching those three score years and ten, rightfully owed me and, as I interpret, what is promised in the Bible. My optimism is strained, but I cannot just lie back and get ready to die. Surely, someone will phone in a solution; maybe there's something we've overlooked; like maybe two pages of the book, the book that must exist somewhere that gives solutions to illnesses such as mine, were stuck together and, when that's noticed, a solution will be there. Yeah, right.

V

*In which a miracle takes place and a new drug
makes me feel better and not as though I am
about to die, but not enough better to
reduce my wish to try an additional drug, which no
one will prescribe for me*

And then the most extraordinary thing happens. You've heard of *deus ex_machina*; well, here is ours! My daughter Annie calls to say that a friend has called her (out of the blue, from New York, at 3:00 AM), having just heard on a CNN broadcast that there is a new, still experimental, drug for my kind of leukemia that is being tested at several medical centers, including UCLA, and that it has been 100% effective—pretty impressive results, I daresay. Annie then finds the specific information on CNN's website and prints it out for us. It's like a Hollywood movie. Even though the number of people in the sample of patients in the study is only thirty-four, I clearly need an entré into this study and this drug.

Next time I'm in to see Charlie, I bring with me the CNN printout and start to talk with him about this miracle drug, STI 571, but I notice very quickly, while I am still talking, that he does not share my enthusiasm and glee. To the contrary, he says that there are always these "miracle" drugs showing up, and unfortunately they don't go anywhere. I point out the success rate claimed in the article, he points out the very small sample. I want to argue that I remember from my statistics classes a long time ago that it is more difficult to get positive results at a significant level from a small sample than from a large one, but what if I am remembering incorrectly? After all, my last statistics course was forty-five years ago. What can I do? My disappointment is, as you might imagine, huge. Certainly he knows his field quite a bit better than I do, so I try to let it slide and my panacea is flushed away (it seems to me that sometimes, I simply cannot express myself adequately without mixing metaphors, so please forgive).

Our next appointment is put off a while because Charlie is going to a hematology conference in New Orleans. When we do get together after he gets back, he tells me that he'd heard about my "miracle" drug at the conference and that the buzz is that it would be well worth pursuing (when he hears it from me or CNN, he doesn't believe it, and I imagine that he didn't tell his buddies at the conference about the problem with this small sample), that I should call the research people at UCLA, that he will email the people he knows there, and that I ought to try to get into Phase II of the research: Interferon failures (this is the first time in my life that I can enjoy being a failure!).

So Diana dials the project's phone number and follows the directions in their message. We do everything they ask: we leave them a message with our phone number, I fax them a brief history of my disease—and then we wait for them to call back. I have no doubt at all that I am the ideal candidate for them, one of those Interferon failures that we know they need for their Phase II sample. There is no doubt that we have done exactly what their message asked us to do, and yet, days pass, we wait, and the telephone does not ring. Surely those people down there know that my life is at stake and yet they don't call back. And not to respond to Charlie's e-mail! Who are these non-empathic, careless people?

After a few days, I realize that I have an ace up my sleeve. A recent friend had been a biggie in the hematology-oncology department down there before he retired up here and, although he is not too enthusiastic about the likelihood of any real effect on the disease by this soon-to-be "*My* Miracle Drug" (in fact, who except me would be?), he certainly feels it's worth a look-see; he is willing to e-mail the people down there about me. He does and, *mirabile dictu*, they call us the next day, and we make arrangements to go down to LA a few days later, to become part of a research protocol, for all practical purposes to partake in a miracle, and to save my life.

Part of what the research people down there say they need from the people up here is a recent bone marrow aspiration and biopsy and we arrange to have that done in Charlie's operation up here. A woman, a nurse practitioner it seems to me, takes Diana and me to an examining room, tells us that she will be doing the biopsy, and that before she starts she would like me to take a little sedative (I'm always impressed now with the word *little* when it comes to things medical!). I tell her that I wouldn't like to do that, that I don't want any sedative, I don't like the feeling that downers leave me with for the rest of the day, that on previous occasions when I've had this procedure, nobody even suggested giving me any sedatives. She says, "Of course they did. They probably didn't mention it specifically, but the procedure is not an easy one and there is no doubt that you will need a sedative." Now, apparently this woman does this all the time. I don't. I have learned that doctors (and nurse practitioners) don't always tell you accurately what they are doing; she knows this as well as I do. But I do know that I've never been given a shot or asked to take a pill before the procedure. I don't like how I am going to feel, but she knows what she's doing, so I'm bullied into finally saying OK and then, after the procedure, I suffer that groggy, post-downer feeling all day long. And I know for sure now after many subsequent biopsies that I simply do not need what she calls a "sedative."

We go down to UCLA for two days. There are interviews, my history is taken several times, blood is drawn (at one point every half hour; I ought to mention that by now I am almost oblivious to needles), a bone marrow aspiration and biopsy are done (remember I just had one done for them per their request the week before, but no matter—I'm glad to give them marrow in exchange for something like a promise of life!). So now I have become part of the research: four miracle pills are brought to me by a nurse while I'm sitting in a busy waiting room, as if to confirm publicly my acceptance into the group, an appointment is set to return in four weeks (it will be once every four weeks for twenty four weeks, then once every twelve weeks for a year, then once every twenty-four weeks) and then I'm back home.

The waiting area is quite a large room, the check-in area on the long wall, directly opposite the entrance, and it's furnished on both sides of the check-in area with living room furniture, everything is wood and upholstery, a soft, country look, the fabric a floral pattern, not quite chintz—no metal, nothing officey here. Partly done jig-saw puzzles cascade around the top of the round, splayed-leg table in the middle of the sitting area to the right of the check-in; it would be homey, but for its ersatz quality (that is, it looks like a hospital area disguised to look like an

English living room) and for the fact that nobody I know would use furniture like this. The only reading material is cancer-oriented magazines and tracts.

The look really is that of a dayroom in a costly private psychiatric facility, except that half the people sitting around (the other half are accompanying family members) look to be sick, fragile, sallow, skinny, and, the give-away, many wearing head coverings. But, whether the décor is successful or not, there was an administrator here who decided at some point that it might be helpful to patients that their contact with Hematology-Oncology be as nonclinical, as comfortable as possible, that it be as homelike as money and taste allow; somebody here thought and cared about what the experience of the patient might be. (You might be interested to know that after several years, the furniture begins to look a bit old, so they refurnish, this time with conventional, not unattractive doctors' waiting room furniture: no more jig saw puzzles, no more chintz, no more down-home. I guess that the original innovator is gone and for those who remain, enough is enough.)

Because of the way the seating is arranged, couches at right angles to each other, wing chairs around a game table, conversation, thus made easy, is constant and cannot be ignored. But while you are there, it's a bit dangerous to open yourself up to conversation with anyone sitting next to you on a sofa or in a wing chair across from you, because once the conversation begins, there is bound to be an outpouring of every turn of events in the history of that person's (or that person's spouse's, parent's, or child's) cancer, and, trust me, if you're feeling at all nervous when you get there, this is not something you want to get into.

Once you check in, after a brief wait, someone calls out your name (first and last names), you are weighed, vital signs are taken, blood is drawn, and if there is an empty examining room (and there usually is) you wait there for the doctor to see you and for the bone marrow stuff to be done. The wait is very short.

Charles Sawyers, the man I deal with most down there, seems tuned in just right, a rarity, I'd thought, in a researcher: he listens, he never talks down, he gives off the feeling that you're an intelligent person, that you're human, and that where you might go on a vacation, for example, is of some interest to him. And everyone else I deal with down there is like that too. It does not distract them that I am a person. And they seem proud of what they are doing, excited about this new drug they're dealing with. It's a pleasure to deal with them and to be part of this enterprise . . . especially if it is going to work.

Now let me tell you, before we go on, about this drug, now called *Gleevec*—a rather disappointing name, I feel—the initial hard *G*, the *vec* at the end, are both quite unpleasant, the joy promised in the first syllable is obviated by the second, and, more to the point, the name means nothing; the drug company had apparently copyrighted the name for a drug they were researching, but ended up not marketing. Such a wonderful drug deserves a regal, sonorous name. Gleevec (you will re member that it was called STI 571 during the initial part of the research and I liked that, at least for its mystery and the wondering it caused) was approved by the FDA for the treatment of CML in May, 2001, after I'd been on it a year and a half, quite a bit earlier than other drugs would have been approved, because the data showed very dramatically a significantly better response to this drug than to the conventional therapy at that time—essentially, Interferon. And much milder side effects to boot!

Here's how Gleevec (the chemical name is *imatinib mesylate*, just in case that sort of thing is interesting to you) works. It blocks the action of the Bcr-Abl tyrosine kinese, the protein produced by the Philadelphia chromosome that I described to you before, and, in so doing, not only stops the increase in CML white cells, but in about half the cases gets rid too of the Philadelphia chromosome (we are not yet sure how this happens, but my idea is that since the Philadelphia chromosome is no longer destructively effective, it gives up the ghost, lies back, and just dies.) Gleevec is the first cancer drug that turns off the signal of the specific cancer causing protein; other cancer drugs have interfered with proteins associated with the cancers—here we are dealing with the cause itself of the cancer! The charm, though, is not only in what it does do; it is also very impressive in what it does not do. That is to say, since the drug is so specifically targeted, it doesn't really impinge on other physiological processes and therefore, for the most part, in most people who've used it, the side effects of Gleevec, unlike those of most other cancer drugs, are usually quite tolerable.

An interesting (to me) aside. Remember that there are not enough new cases of CML to make R&D on CML drugs economically worthwhile. Well, once the CML community got wind that there was a drug which seemed likely to be useful in the treatment of the disease and that Novartis, the company that makes the drug, for economic reasons, was very likely not going to pursue its development, the company was inundated with e-mails, begging, insisting, threatening that it continue pursuing the drug's development. This inundation was sufficiently thunderous that the company succumbed, developed, and here we are! This is one of the early uses of the Internet for political ends.

A particular joy for me about going down to UCLA and being in this project is the parking situation there. You have to take pleasure where you can find it. I drive into their garage, which is surprisingly cleaner and better lighted than most garages in my experience, pay my five dollars (it has now gone up to eight dollars), go to the oncology department and they do their thing. The visit over, the oncology people give me a chit and when I leave the garage, I give the chit to the attendant and he gives me back the five dollars I paid. I'm spending money on airfare and a rental car, yet I'm thrilled to get the five dollars back. Speaking about airfare, let me just mention that when I entered the project, United's fare for a round trip, coming back on the same day, was $116; four years later it was $340 (I think that because I come back on the same day their computers have begun to assume that I am a business man and that my business will pay the airfare, so up it goes)—the price has almost tripled in five years. I won't take on the airlines, here; maybe later—my focus now is medicine, but I had to let you know. Maybe at another time I could do an airline memoir, because, trust me, there too I could fill a book.

Since I've mentioned airlines, I would like, at the risk of seeming peevish, a quality I would stoutly disavow, to comment on some of the similarities between the airlines and the medical establishment. Obviously you rely on each to get you where you'd like to go, and most of the time they get you there, but it all has to take place on their terms. And when they don't get you there, it's very big bad news. There is enough attitude in each enterprise to disarm the most intrepid. And each blames outside forces (litigation and thus insurance in one, gas prices and unions in the other) to justify their prices. Seats in each are not comfortable and it's hard to resist the feeling, dealing with each, that everything is set up for the staff's convenience.

An additional thing that makes the garage so wonderful is a comparison with the garage at the medical center up here. The one up here is not so spic-and-span clean nor so well lighted and despite all the signs on my favorite floor (the top floor—my favorite, because from the top floor you can drive directly to the street, from any other floor you have to wind your way down spiraling past all the floors below you in this eight story garage) that say "Small cars only," the place is full of SUV's; they make parking very tight, and since the lanes are pretty narrow and the SUV's stick out so far, it's hard to get out of a space and navigate down the lanes (though it is rather a kick to watch the SUV's struggle to get out of their spaces).

One more interesting sidelight about the medical center garages: up here it's two dollars for the first hour, but if you drive out in less than twenty minutes, it's free. There was a long period of time when I was going in weekly just to have blood drawn for the research and I would have to deal with the terrible, but very exciting, tension of parking, then taking one elevator to get out of the garage, then a second elevator to get to the hematology clinic, then checking in at the clinic, and waiting for the lab people to call me, and then working my way all the way back to the car and out as the minutes ticked away. On a very good day, I could do it in just under twenty minutes, but usually it was just over twenty minutes and I was stuck. There aren't a lot of good days. It's not the money; two dollars is just two dollars, even for me, a depression boy. It's whether you win or lose—and there's no way for me to view this enterprise (and, I'm afraid, so many others) as anything other than a contest. As always, you win some, you lose some. But when you win, when the parking has been free, the thrill is great.

Another remarkable thing down there is the piano music. In the main, very busy lobby of the building that houses the oncology clinic, there is a piano, and from time to time, it seems unpredictable and unscheduled, a man plays standards. Since the building is, I think, an outpatient facility, people do what waiting they need to do in clinic waiting rooms, not in the main lobby. There are, then, at most, a handful of people sitting around in the lobby; there are many people (with or without a myriad of attachments signifying illness) going through the lobby, scurrying to and from appointments, to and from the lab and the pharmacy, in and out of the store that sells snacks and periodicals, the audience is less like that of a geriatric center than that at Nordstrom. Yet there he is, when he is there, playing his heart out. One asks oneself, "Who is that man playing for," and the very heartening answer is, "He plays for thee—however transient your attention might be." In addition to the nostalgic pleasure of the music, it is the oddity of the situation, the Fellini quality, and that its presence is unpredictable that give it its special pleasure.

I'm on four pills of Gleevec every morning (at first, two hours after breakfast, i.e., on an empty stomach, and, as likely as not, I spend the day with varying degrees of nausea; then, after eight weeks, the data support the notion that the medicine is metabolized equally well with or without food, so the pills are taken with breakfast and I can feel pretty good all day long) and in fewer than eight weeks my blood counts are fine, the white counts are well within the normal range (this is called *hematologically* clear), and after 24 weeks, no Philadelphia chromosome is evident in my marrow (this is called *cytologically* clear), even by a

89

FISH test. (Let me simplify: let's say a regular biopsy exam looks at 20 cells, a FISH test looks at 100 cells, and a *PCR* at ten thousand). Here's the place where the music swells to signify a miracle, for me a true miracle.

On the *PCR*, initiated routinely after I'd been in the project two years, there is still a very small trace of this chromosomal anomaly—the Philadelphia chromosome—no one knows why, the research indicates that there seems to be no difference in what happens with the disease, at least so far, in this short haul, between those who get rid of the Philadelphia chromosome completely and people like me who retain an infinitesimally small amount, and, after a few years now, the number has not begun to increase nor the cells to mutate. As a matter of fact, the most recent research indicates that I'm probably in very good shape for a long time.

It is, for me, indeed a miracle drug! I am soaring! I am a very lucky man. A small percentage of subjects in the project have not been responsive to the drug, a few others have intolerable side effects; in another small percent, the chromosome mutates and new problems occur, not a good feeling if that happens to you (even then, fortunately, the researchers have produced new drugs that zap the mutations). I know, as they say, twenty-four/seven, how lucky and grateful I am.

I remain in the project six years, going down to LA every twenty-four weeks; the drug company still requiring bone marrow biopsies for their research each time I'm there, but after a while decides that they will no longer pay for them. So I continue doing it, my insurance pays for the procedure even though the drug company demands it (I guess that in this day and age you need good insurance to be a guinea pig), and although my insurance would pay for the Gleevec, since the FDA approved it early, the project gives me a 24 week supply of capsules to take home (Novartis, through my local drug store, would be charging me $14,400 for the package), when I'm down there every twenty four weeks. So the insurance company is doing better financially paying for the biopsies (they end up a lot cheaper than the drug, since they take place only every six months). Everybody wins!

While I am on the subject of insurance, I need to say that Medicare plus my secondary insurance are wonderful plans and should be what everybody in this country has: I pay for nothing except small co-payments on medicine. I am one of those very fortunate people who do not have to worry about medical costs. Because of that, I'm afraid, I have become somewhat irresponsible, in that I rarely look at bills. There are exceptions, however: when a medical bill comes from someone whose name on the return address is not familiar, then I look. These are rarely mistakes; sometimes the sender is part of a team and the name simply went by me and sometimes the bills are for encounters that happened so long ago that I've forgotten the name. I recently was sent a bill for a procedure that took place two weeks less than a year and a half before the date of the bill's delivery.

While this sort of thing is not frequent, this is not the first time I've gotten a bill that was more than a year old, and I get to wonder how these doctors subsist during the year that their bills are not sent out. I guess that that is something I should not be concerned about, but I find this kind of rumination distracting and perhaps amusing. When I call the office where the bill originates, they explain, for example, that they did not have my insurance information, as though that explains a year and a half delay in billing. Why this might be true is a mystery to me since, immediately upon my entering a medical office for the first time, I am asked for my insurance cards—before the outside door closes, before I can catch my breath. But you have to wonder anyway, if they need information from me they have my address (they did, after all, use it finally to send me the bill) and my phone number is in the book; they could certainly have contacted me months and months ago. So I then become quite a little concerned about what else goes wrong in that office: are test results on the basis of which the diagnoses are made really mine and are they correct, could I have somebody else's results, for example, and thus his/her diagnosis? These worries clearly take my mind off my real problems.

The FDA approved the drug early, because of the astounding clarity of the very positive results in Phases I and II of the research—despite the small initial sample!—and therefore my insurance would cover the expense of the drug (it's $2400 a month—remember, there aren't a lot of customers to pay for all that R&D, so the cost goes up; why the specific figure $2400?—we think that the company decided to charge what people had been paying for Interferon, which as you remember was the only available but not very effective drug for CML in the past). When the FDA approved the drug, the researchers gave me the choice of stopping or continuing. If I left the study, I would not have to go down to LA when I don't feel like it, and I would save on air fare and car rental, My answer is that I stay because of the romantic notion that they saved my life and I owe them. A little romanticism surely is appropriate here! There is also for me, the fact, I am a little embarrassed to admit, that I feel myself a pioneer, I'm involved in a project that is going to save many lives, partly because of my involvement. It's a great feeling! And *we* are teaching other cancer researchers an approach to the field that has worked so well here. It all makes me feel terrific, a do-gooder and very studly.

But miracles too have their costs apparently and, while not even close to devastating, there are some side effects. Common are fatigue (the UCLA folks keep wanting to convince me that mine very likely has its roots elsewhere, like my age or some other pill I'm on, but I know it's the drug and from the web site I see that everyone on the drug has the same complaint), muscle cramps (the first week I wake up screaming one night from the pain in my calf; that and cramps elsewhere continue, though the screaming has mostly abated), edema (mine, fortunately is restricted to puffiness around my eyes—I have not gotten myself to use *Preparation H* on my eyelids; it does, I'm told with some logic, for eyelids what it's supposed to do for hemorrhoids, which is what the people on the web site of those with the disease suggest. Ice works some, but frankly it is too uncomfortable on my eyelids to make it a habit), and a rash (mine, consistent with the comments of the UCLA people when they looked at it, turned out to be caused by something else).

The sleepiness is a pain in the neck, but maybe the research people are right and mine is not from Gleevec. At any rate, I ask every doctor I'm involved with to help me with the fatigue: "My hemoglobin is lower than normal, I'm tired all the time, I'm anemic, wouldn't it make sense for me to be on *Procrit*?" and everyone of them responds the same way: "Your hemoglobin is not that low; it's just below normal limits and you would not be considered anemic, maybe you're tired because of your age, Procrit is too expensive, and your hemoglobin is not low enough for

your insurance to justify covering the cost of the drug. No!"
So I nap every day and complain less.

And just what is this Procrit that I keep asking for? They
don't really tell you on the abundant TV commercials, do
they? They just indicate that it's good to take in order to
up your energy while you are taking cancer-related drugs,
so that you can play energetically with your grandchildren.
Nor do they mention in the ubiquitous commercials
(ubiquitous, that is, if you are a channel surfer) that it has
to be injected. *Procrit* is, in fact, a manufactured form of
Erythropoietin (also called, I think affectionately, *Epo*).
Just like the stuff your kidneys produce, it stimulates the
production of red cells from bone marrow. It is a colorless
liquid that is injected weekly and essentially works the
same as kidney-produced Erythropoietin to promote the
production of red cells.

VI

*In which two new medical problems arise,
one easily dealt with, the other possibly frightening,
both of which I manage with some ultimate success,
even while my wife and I deal with an alarming
situation of hers.*

I wasn't going to bother you with the story of my glaucoma, mostly because it seemed minor, I never experienced any symptoms or problems from the disease, and because it's working out fine, with very little aggravation. It didn't occupy a great deal of time and attention. But since my intention here is to build as complete a picture as I can, here goes.

In the middle of this barrage of medical involvements, I decide that I need new glasses, but I haven't had an eye exam in a long time. I go to an ophthalmologist I've not seen before; Diana has been seeing him for years and likes him. In the waiting room are beautiful magazines about photography and about tribal art, the women at the reception desk are very attractive and personable, so I'm feeling good about this.

I'm called into an examining room, a little ritual goes on with techs and those hard plastic eye patch paddles, then the ophthalmologist himself comes in, introduces himself with a firm handshake, and we begin. He seems quite open, he responds appropriately to questions about himself, apparently willing to let me know him, and he talks about what he is seeing as the exam moves along. He checks everything out and says to me at the end that while my "pressures" are not significantly above normal, looking at my optic nerve, there is good reason to suspect glaucoma. I'm there for a refraction for glasses and he tells me, out of the blue, that I have glaucoma! Two cancers and a hiatal hernia are apparently not enough for me; I am going blind too? That's not exactly what I woke up hoping for this morning!

This interaction is completely absurd to me; I do not want to listen to what he is saying. Enough already! But it would not look good if I just upped and left the office, so I'm stuck. He is, after all, not only engaging, but he also talks to me like an adult, as though I might be able to understand his logic. He does not talk down. Yet, since, for me, glaucoma is defined as high pressures, I don't get this at all. I tell him that even as a youngster, like when I was in the army, my retinas, my optic nerves, my maculae (it's true, too, but I guess I'm trying to impress him with the specialized vocabulary) have taken doctors aback at first, and that that millisecond response by them used to scare me. I'll use anything to dissuade him from this very rash diagnosis. I tell him about my optometrist, who always checks my retinas, and that when I saw him last, maybe eighteen months ago, he did not indicate that there were any problems. He says he'll call him and then will get back to me. He also says, almost as an after-thought, that I don't need new glasses. My agenda is glasses and his is glaucoma. Serves me right, I guess, for eschewing my optometrist this time and seeing an ophthalmologist. Forget it! I'm out of there.

Later that day, he calls me from his car, on his cell phone—this in an era when cell phones are not so rife as they are today—to tell me through the traffic sounds that he called my optometrist and that the optometrist checked his records and found no indication of a problem, but that he, the ophthalmologist, still feels that the situation should be monitored and taken seriously. It's the calling from the car that provides me with an excuse; is, business transacted with me on a cell-phone rarely is going to fill me with glee. There could not be a better excuse for me not to call his office for a follow-up appointment, never really to contact him again. And, perhaps more to the point, for me, my optometrist, the fellow I eschewed for this, is not chopped liver; why should I believe a new acquaintance over an old one? And as I am sure you will agree I have enough diagnoses without this one. So I use my justifications and I don't call.

Well, I manage to put it off a year, expecting that, during that year, things will somehow align differently, he will forget about this glaucoma nonsense, and we will start afresh, on a new slate. A year later (apparently this thing is much on my mind while I'm doing nothing about it), I'm feeling a little funny about the whole glaucoma business—surely the fellow is not simply making this up; and he has never over-diagnosed Diana. So, very ambivalently, I make an appointment to see him. He checks out my eyes with all that nifty apparatus and tells me exactly what he'd said the first time. In addition, he wants me to do a visual fields test.

So I go in for the test, it's all very casual, the young woman tells me that, with my head immobile in the apparatus, I am to focus on a spot in the center, and that I will see dots of light flashing all over, and each time that

I do I am to press a button. The task seems impossible to me. How do you see flashes when your looking at one spot, are all the flashes the same size, could there be several in a row near the same area?—but I go along and finish. I have the feeling that my button pressing is close to arbitrary and that nothing meaningful can come out of this foolish exercise. But I go back to see the doctor a few days later and he shows me the computer image of how my optic nerve is responding and it looks just like what he had predicted.

I don't like this situation at all, but the computer image knocks out any possibility for my denial, and this time I go along, I ask questions, he answers and gives numbers, he prescribes eye drops, I then do the drops nightly, and now, for a couple of years, he likes the new very stable numbers and is happier with my optic nerves. There is something to be said for making these fellows happy. I see him now every three months.

Early in our contacts, he notices in the records that I have CML (Chronic Melogenous Leukemia, remember?) and asks if I am on Gleevec. I tell him my story briefly and he is very interested because a relative of his was recently diagnosed with CML and is on Gleevec. He asks questions about it, the research, my side effects, how I handle things, and I become an expert to him. He tells me stories about his relative. A little role reversal perhaps, and though he begins the CML conversation each time a little shyly, a little tenuously, there seems very little discomfort with the fact that each of us treats the other as human, each with his own area of expertise. I know by his manner, by his attention, that he is interested in me and that if it were not CML and Gleevec, our discourse would be on a different subject. There is some indication that he forgets about me between contacts, but when he looks in my file his ideas about me start in again, so that at least for the time we are together, there is this interaction and reciprocity. That is enough for me. That's all I'm asking for.

There really is not too much to say about my prostate cancer, diagnosed two and a half years after the leukemia and the kidney cancer. Let me explain first that the prostate is a walnut sized, doughnut shaped cluster of glands, at the bottom of the bladder, near the base of the penis. Increases in its size and shape can often be detected by a digital rectal exam.

I go in for a regular annual physical again—maybe that's my problem: without the physicals the disease is not diagnosed and maybe without the diagnosis it doesn't exist; maybe it's like a tree falling in the forest (although once when I explained this iatrogenic view of all disease to a psychiatrist friend of mine, his face darkened, he asked if I really believed what I was saying, and I knew he was afraid I was going crazy); in the blood work they find that my *PSA*, usually about one, is a little over five.

PSA (Prostate Specific Antigen) is produced in the prostate and is secreted by the prostate into semen; it prevents coagulation of semen. Normally small amounts leak into the bloodstream. If there is cancer in the prostate, the ducts that normally secrete PSA into the urethra get clogged; thus more PSA leaks out into the bloodstream.

As is my wont, I decide to do nothing for a while, to watch it. OK, maybe not even to watch it—to ignore it. My newly acquired urologist (acquired because of my new PSA figure) may be nervous about this, but he is, at least verbally, respectful of my decision. But he wants to see me in a few months and at this second contact my PSA is up another point and even I can't put off dealing much longer.

So the urologist does a biopsy of my prostate. I've put up with many uncomfortable procedures—remember, I'm the guy who has no qualms about bone marrow biopsies!—but never have I even contemplated the possibility of anything quite so uncomfortable, so humiliating as this! For the biopsy, I'm on a table on my side, my ass exposed, he puts some contraption up my ass that allows him not only to feel the prostate, but to cut through the intestinal wall in order to sample several very small pieces of the prostate; every time the instrument cuts, and I think it does four, there is a loud click (at least to me it is thunderous) and it hurts! It is the anticipation of the clicks, which, after the first one, sound even louder to me, that contributes to my general horror and to a soreness in every muscle in my body from the tension. I leave the office a far different person, older and, I think, wiser than when I went in!

He tells me, by the way, that very likely there will be blood in my urine for a few days. Had I known that before, I would have tried to refuse the biopsy (in the same way, I suppose, that I try to refuse just about everything else), because blood in my urine does not sit well with me. It gives me the creeps and there is no way that I can avoid seeing it when I urinate—if I don't look, I might miss the bowl, and perhaps more important, I won't know if the bleeding has stopped. So for a while, in addition to everything else going on with me, I am grossed out and frightened every time I urinate. It's not that I urinate pink, which I think would have been even less tolerable for me than the little red drops at the beginning and the end, floating in the bowl. I do not like what I see at all, but I cannot quite put my finger on what is so disturbing! I think it may be that here is specific, concrete evidence that something is wrong with me internally, and yet there is nothing I can do about it; it is beyond the realm of band-aids or pressure—I am a passive witness to something in me, far beyond my control.

In relation to the bleeding, he tells me that if it doesn't stop in a week, I should call him. So after seven days of urinary dread, I call to tell him that the bleeding is continuing. He comments that that's OK, that happens, and that I ought to give it another week and, if it hasn't stopped by then, to get in touch with him. Am I missing something? Now my fantasy is that for the rest of my life I will be calling him weekly and each time he will put me off for a week. Not to worry! The bleeding does stop in a few days.

A few days after the biopsy (but before the bleeding has stopped), he calls to tell me that the results are positive. Again, I've got the big C! I'm batting 1000. Every time something is suspected, I've got it! (Three times in two and a half years! Is this a record? What is the prize? Who gives it out?). Analogies to Job might now be in order.

Before I continue, I ought to tell you a little about prostate cancer and its treatment. There are two things to keep in mind:

1. for the most part, prostate cancer in an old man's disease (80% of prostate cancer cases occur in men over 65—when people died younger, it was rarely seen);

2. in most European countries, very little is done about prostate cancer, because generally the disease progresses more slowly than our age does (as a matter of fact 80% of men over eighty have some degree of prostate cancer) and we die of something else—the problem here is that that is not always true and a significant number of people do die of this cancer and of problems related to

it—cancer of the prostate is the leading cause of cancer deaths among non-smoking American men.

There are essentially three kinds of treatments for prostate cancer: radical surgery, radiation, and waiting and watching. There are two kinds of radiation: external radiation (radiation therapy daily for six weeks—every day! six weeks!) and *brachitherapy* (from the Greek for *near*). *Brachitherapy* is a procedure that deposits radioactive seeds (tiny pellets, filled in my case, with radioactive iodine) into the prostate, injected through the perineum, based on a 3-D model of the prostate constructed previously.

I'm offered these choices by the head of radiation therapy to whom I have been sent by my urologist. For me, it's great that the choice is mine: I feel that they're treating me like an adult, and also I can see myself as more in control of what's happening to me. The problem is that I have almost no basis for making a choice: a twenty minute conversation here in the office and some very cursory reading on the Internet—so actually my decision is based on little more than which kind of intervention will cause me the least inconvenience.

I choose brachitherapy, the main reason being that it is a one time procedure (daily radiation for six weeks, being brought so regularly, so directly, so concretely, so frequently, and for six weeks yet, in contact with the definiteness of my latest cancer gives me the heebie-jeebies), non-invasive compared to surgery and with many fewer side effects, and with just about the same positive results.

When I suggest to him that seeding, *brachitherapy*, sounds like the most reasonable way for me to proceed, he nods and asks if we'd like to meet the doctor in charge of the program. I know that *in charge* means that this doctor is the only one who does this procedure there, so I say, "Sure," he makes the phone call, and tells us that the doctor will be right over.

There is a scene in *From Here to Eternity*, the first time you see Deborah Kerr, she is walking. swinging her purse, and the music accompanying the walk signals to us her perhaps brazen sexuality (as opposed to Ms. Kerr's reticence in the previous roles by which we have come to known her). The same sort of thing happens when my new radiologist enters, preceded by the staccato clicking of her heels on the floor (the music swelling in our heads): a very attractive woman in her middle 30's, short black skirt, surprisingly high heels, very dark hair, red, very red lipstick, and very red polish on long nails, the whole picture just this glorious side of cheap. I think the other things I remember about her attire and her manner I'd better not mention since they are very likely things I've added in my fantasy over the last couple of years (having been thoroughly affected by *To Have and Have Not*, as an eighth grader, but I don't think she asked me for a light). She is wonderful and dramatic to look at, and I am sure I've made the right choice. Glamour and my prostate! A combination to contemplate!

We talk about the procedure and make an appointment for her to take measurements of my prostate; those measurements will then be sent to a group in Seattle (why Seattle?) that will construct a model and we will then be able to do the seeding a few weeks later, using the model as a guide. I come for the measurement session and do what she asks. That is to say, almost naked, I'm lying on my back on a table, my ankles in stirrups, as I recall the lighting is quite low, she's got some instrument up my ass (though this time it manages to be somehow much less degrading and uncomfortable than the biopsy), moving it around some, and she is recording whatever it's measuring, all this with a certain amount of casualness on her part and exchanged pleasantries. In the middle of this, the head guy, the one I'd met on my previous visit and who had given me the choices, waltzes in to see how things are going. In the middle of this most private and, at the same time, I must acknowledge, most intimate experience, he doesn't even knock; and then he walks over to me to say hello and to ask how I'm doing. The way I remember it, he even wants to shake my hand!

Anyway the thing gets measured, I imagine that the model gets constructed, and a couple of weeks later we are all ready for the seeding. Despite some O.R. costumery, my radiologist is able to communicate the same red lipsticky thing that she'd done during our previous encounters. The operating room is getting a little crowded, but it's all very congenial—it reminds me of the lobby of a synagogue during Yom Kippur services, small groups, everyone chatting, but everything's in hushed tones, as though not to disturb the service.

My urologist is there and he tells me that he thinks that I did right by choosing the seeding over the other kind of radiation (Look. I like my urologist a lot. He is respectful and open. But what is this: a test of my ability to choose a medical procedure on the basis of virtually no knowledge? If, as it turns out, he thinks one approach better than another, why didn't he advise me before I had to decide?—I get my information, after all, from the Internet, his sources are likely more rounded and with fewer holes—what would he have said if I'd made another choice; on the other hand, we know by now, don't we, that if he had given me advice, I would probably have resented that too—what is a doctor to do?); but when I tell him that I am flying to Aspen the following morning to spend the week-end with Diana who is there for a two week workshop, he comes very close to forbidding it! (Maybe he should have. The consequences of post-brachitherapy and the high altitude of the Rockies are not entirely pleasant. The details I will not go into, except to say that more time is spent in the bathroom than in bed or anywhere else).

The two things most endearing to me about the procedure itself are:

1. there is a group of people clustered near my head during the procedure (I can't imagine and am not told what their function might be), and that gives me people to talk with while the procedure is going on at the other end of me, and

2. a physicist is present; I find this particularly exciting, offbeat, modern, even surreal—even though I don't know quite what he is doing there.

The procedure ends and everyone is happy, even though I am told to return a few days later for an x-ray. to see if any of these radioactive seeds got into my lungs (It turns out that one did. "Next time you have an x-ray," she says, "make sure you tell them to expect it!"). She tells me to email her if any problems arise. She also tells me to be careful around children, not to hold any child on my now radioactive lap.

After a couple of days, I e-mail her, as she has instructed me, to tell her that my continuing terrible diarrhea awakens me many times during the night. Her response is that she's not heard of that before and doesn't know what to suggest. Period! Well, then, find out! She is the doctor! She is apparently without any helpful information unless the thing sounds specifically like it belongs within her specialty, even though the organ currently in question is very close to the organ she'd been tampering with. The problem began immediately after a procedure done by a doctor I have had good feelings for and she won't even make the effort to check things out, if it doesn't sound to her like a problem relating to the seeding itself. From her point of view my diarrhea, whenever it may have started, relates to a different organ system, so forget it. This despite our knowledge that the area radiated is pretty close to the bowel.

Now catch this. I recently met a man who had had similar treatment for prostate cancer. He told me that he had terrible diarrhea for more than six months after the treatment. When he spoke to his radiologist about this, he was told that there was certainly no relationship between these symptoms and the procedure and that he ought to follow up on the diarrhea with his internist. I would suggest a pattern here, but it gets even better. Sometime later, after many months, the diarrhea finally gone, he ran into someone he knew who had the same experience and the same denial of possible relationship. All of us with different doctors telling us the same cop-out story. Three out of three. Can we consider this a finding?

By the way, my PSA went down rather quickly to where it had been before and has stayed there. This happy result has not tempered my urologist's eagerness to do me frequent rectal examinations. I tried arguing that so long as my PSA stays where it is, especially since it was a rise in PSA that signaled the problem and not a rectal examination—those were always negative, there is good reason to assume no problem; and especially since there was no change in the feel of my prostate through a rectal exam at the time the diagnosis was made. But he is adamant about the need for a rectal examination (either he can bill Medicare for it or it's his thing—I don't know and ultimately what difference does it make), he is generally very nice to me, by now I've gotten used to the experience, so I usually let him. It's important to him, so what the hell, why not! I'm easy.

Now, here I've told you the story of my prostate cancer as though nothing else were going on in my world, but that gives too simple a picture of my experience. So I'll back up a little time-wise, in order to give you some context. Around the time that I am trying to decide what kind of treatment to choose for my prostate cancer, Diana notices a small lump in her right breast. Holy shit! We are the house of Atreus, but what did we do wrong? Where is our hubris?

Terrifying, of course, for any woman (or man, for that matter; remember that Bill, Diana's first husband, died from the consequences of breast cancer), but especially difficult in this case, because fourteen years before, while we were courting, Diana noticed a lump in the same breast, and eventually had a lumpectomy and then was treated with radiation. At that time, it seems that two pathologists differed about whether or not a biopsy indicated that it was malignant; but the surgery was done (better safe than sorry), margins were what they were supposed to be and there seemed to be no lymph node involvement. Diana followed up with mammograms (which, however, were negative both before the episode fourteen years ago and this new one) and saw the breast surgeon routinely for a number of years after the surgery. After fourteen years, you feel that you can breathe easy about yourself and worry instead about your husband. No such luck! Oh, fickle finger of fate!

So she calls Ernie Rosenbaum (he seems to be our on-call cancer guy, the first level of our very own cancer triage) and we go in to see him. He examines her, schedules a bunch of tests and says that he thinks that this is not a recurrence, but rather a new primary lesion. If you are going to have cancer, it's better to have a new one, because if it's the same as the old one, it means that the surgery and radiation did not get all of it and cells have been lying around for this long, maybe by now all over the place and God knows how to locate them.

I don't know whether to think of our situation as four cancers in one couple in three years or five cancers in fourteen years. I think the former is the more impressive statement and I'll stick with it.

Imagine the emotional climate in our household: roles are reversed, for the moment, and I am again the caretaker I'd been used to being (somehow, my prostate has taken a back seat to her breast for now); there arise the questions of how and when this plague of cancers of ours will end, what do they want from us? and most important, the terrible anxiety of will she be all right (the doctors seem sanguine and give assurance, but . . .). Our roller coaster keeps speeding along! Crazed though all this makes me, I am a good deal more comfortable worrying about Diana, than having Diana worried about me and I think I do a little better in this role.

Ernie refers her back to her old surgeon, a plain spoken man, whose attitudes and values are clear, and whose scorn for the practice of academic medicine (that is, in hospitals connected with medical schools) is always entertaining. He tells us that in a breast where there is scar tissue from previous surgery, a lumpectomy is impossible, that a mastectomy is the only choice. It is decided in conjunction with Ernie's group to put the surgery off a couple of weeks in order to get back slides of the first tumor, slides that are now stored in Washington, for comparison.

This two-week hiatus is good for Diana, because she had planned on (and paid for) a two-week watercolor workshop in Colorado, beginning like right now. So she goes off to Colorado and I remain at home, where, one week from now, my brachitherapy is to take place. Ruthie will be available to drive me in for the procedure, wait around, and take me home. In the meanwhile, for about a week, I will be the administrator of Diana's pre-surgery: I will handle the papers, phone calls, and faxes to insure that the academics get their slides, and all that administration and busy-work is good for me, because it lessens the likelihood of my obsessing about dark things. The surgeon is amused by all this turmoil, since, with or without the slides, he is going to do the surgery we discussed. Now everyone is glad that Diana, in Colorado, has something productive to keep her busy and away from obsessing about her tumor and surgery.

The old slides finally get here and when they are compared with the recent biopsy, the cells are indeed different. It is definitely a new primary lesion and I give the go-ahead to the surgeon (and the plastic surgeon, who complains that he really should have more time to confer with Diana before the surgery) to set up the surgery for a few days after the Saturday that Diana returns. Meanwhile I get seeded, go to Colorado for the weekend, where Diana signs necessary papers for me to bring back to the principal physicians, and I come home to await Diana's return and her surgery.

She's back on the following Saturday and on Monday has an appointment with the plastic surgeon who will accompany her surgeon in the OR on Tuesday. He is still complaining that he should have more time with her, but they discuss a variety of reconstruction possibilities (from nothing at all to very elaborate tissue-grafting) and, since the surgery is a day away, there's not a lot of time for obsessing; Diana has to choose, on the spot, which she prefers—like picking an ice cream flavor. She chooses the option that is just one step above nothing: virtually a small water balloon, and everything is set for the next day.

Everything goes as planned: a "simple" mastectomy (no need to remove axillary tissue) and a "simple" reconstruction, somewhat disappointing to Diana: a perky right breast and a seventy year old left breast. Follow-up visits are problem-free and we go on with our lives: that is, two weeks after her surgery we go for a planned weekend to the Oregon Shakespeare Festival (six plays in four days, but we still manage naps) and we go on our planned Sicily trip six weeks later, despite the intervention of 9-11, which took place about three weeks post-surgery, a day after our return from Oregon, and a month before we leave for Sicily. Nobody can accuse us of allowing health issues or international calamities to interfere with plans we've made!

Oh, and here's something that may be worth thinking about. Bill had breast cancer; Diana has breast cancer (twice). Sandra had a blood-related cancer (Hodgkin's Disease); I have a blood-related cancer (CML). The pattern is too compelling. You've got to wonder what the fates have in mind here?

Now I have to tell you the truth: I'm beginning to feel a little like a nudnick, kvetching about all these medical issues. It's bad enough that I have all these diagnoses that I am laying on you, but that so much of what I encounter medically I perceive as an injustice, or poorly thought through, or non-empathic or, what can I say, stupid, can be read as something of a pain in the neck. So if I'm beginning to sound like a nudnik to you too, let me make a suggestion: take a break from your reading, do some yard work, maybe go to a ball game, watch a little television, whatever you find distracting, and then come back to this refreshed. You are not going to want to miss some of my adventures that are coming up.

VII

*In which I have much frustration in attempting to
resolve pains in my legs, and I learn
during resolution of that pain that my blood isn't
what it used to be.*

I have neglected to mention this until now, fearing
that your reaction might be, "Enough already with your
kvetching." But here it is now. For years I have been having
pain down both calves when I walk more than a couple of
blocks. Richard has consistently had trouble feeling a pulse
especially in my left foot. In her old age my mother had
serious vascular problems that led to toe amputations, and
those genes do tend to do a number on us. Now a new
problem arises.

I had a fall in Pompeii (just prior to arriving in Sicily)
when, in a very narrow corridor, with very uneven flooring,
I hear what sounds like a horde of German tourists bearing
down on us, their voices and footsteps reverberating off the
walls in these narrow, ancient passageways; my delusional
expectation of the *Horst Wessel Song* provokes in me some
confusion and anxiety (please forgive my stereotyping and
what seems like an inability to forgive; it's not purposeful,
the place is dark and spooky, Conrad Veidt loomed large in
my childhood and some rationality goes out the window),
I lose my footing, career off one wall, then another, and

land, my arm outstretched, on my hand, I have a terrible pain in my right wrist and down my left leg, this on top of the usual problems. And none of it goes away after months. So Richard refers me first to a vascular surgeon.

I have a feeling when we get to the vascular guy's office that this it is not going to be good. First there is a certain amount of disorder and confusion among the women who work in the office—it's hard to articulate just what it is, but the feeling is like doing their nails is the most important part of their job (even though they are not really doing their nails at this exact moment) and this leads to an expectation that they will fail to connect us with the doctor. This quick impression, however, is belied and we are taken to a very nicely furnished room with lots of wood (it's more an office than an examining room) and it is there, when the doctor comes in, that the more important cues to my prognostication show up. Not only is the doctor very short, but he is all dressed up: a dark suit, nifty shirt and tie, and he displays considerable hauteur (he talks like reformed rabbis used to: as close to Oxford speech as an American might get away with)—and none of this compensates for his problems with height.

There is no way he can know what I am thinking, but I very quickly pick up a need of his to keep me in my place and to speak with great authority, and his smile, close to a sneer, never leaves his face. I don't discount the possibility that it may be something in my manner that he is reacting to, but I am not aware of anything I might be doing. What I am aware of, though it is subtle, it is hard to miss, is his condescension. He asks about what is going on, I tell him about Pompeii and my mother and Richard's problem with my pulse. He has me take off my shoes and socks, feels around both feet and ankles and says with a surprising

113

degree of certainty (and, of course, a smile—or do I call it a sneer?) that there is no problem with my pulses, that my problem is not vascular. This evaluation of his is very fast, it's very definite, and very dismissive. We thank him and, bewildered, leave the office.

My feeling is that he just doesn't like me, that he is disdainful of me and I hate that. What did I ever do to him? I know from many conversations with many others, that, in general, people put a lot of stock in having their doctors like them; it's like if the doctor likes them, he/she will take more care with them—if he/she doesn't like them, watch out. We all suspect that this is very likely not true, but in matters relating to our own medical care, as you may have noticed, we are not always rational. Here's a little story. A year after Sandra died, her oncologist, a rather young man with whom I had an easy, pleasant relationship, invites me to a party at his home and I go. At the party, very prominent in my eyes is the doctor who ran the ICU where Sandra spent her last few weeks. Of course, at that time, he and I had a lot of contact. I approach him at the party and very quickly realize that, even after I say my name, he has no idea who I am. I am shocked: my experiences in the hospital were so extraordinarily important to me, how could they have been otherwise for him? This experience is so painful to me that I have to leave the party quite early, unable to consider the number of equally attractive families he has very likely dealt with since I saw him last. The arrogance of my expectation and of my need to remain in his consciousness and in his heart embarrasses me now—but there it is. I had to feel at the time when she was so sick that we were special, that the doctors loved us and would get us through, and that almost delusional idea lingers.

Now, back. OK. Let's cut this vascular fellow some slack—after all, my presenting complaint (the pain down my left leg) turns out, we learn later, to be neurological and not vascular. But how do I deal with his saying that there is no problem with the pulses in my feet? We have learned since that visit that there is blockage in an abdominal artery and in both femoral arteries (the left one being almost entirely closed), so the blood supply down there, at my feet, is going to be pretty meager and, alas, not just happily pulsing along. How can I justify this error of his?

The strangeness of his denial of what I know is true about me reminds me of the time we took Annie, six months old, after we had moved to a different city, to a new pediatrician. He was adamant that we buy her, as soon as possible, shoes (I forget the brand). I said that I didn't understand, since she certainly did not seem close to walking. He did not explain, he simply repeated his statement that it was important, and Sandra and I, very young and unlikely to defy authority (the sixties were just around the corner), went out and bought the shoes and had her wear them. For what? The soles of her feet didn't touch the floor for months. Maybe he owned stock in the shoe company.

The dismissal by this vascular surgeon leads to a neurosurgical consult. The neurosurgeon's office is chaotic. The feeling is that he has just moved in and the office is not yet ready to be open. There are too many people in the waiting room; inside the office suite itself, beyond the waiting room, in the hallway, there are boxes against the wall; and the receptionist, a middle aged Russian woman, seems to have bitten off far more than she can chew and to be absolutely without a clue about what is going on in that waiting room. I feel like I ought to pitch in and help straighten things out—remember I ran outpatient facilities! But the neurosurgeon himself, rather a young man, with Hollywood good looks (kind of a Van Johnson feel to him), and wearing an unusually brown suit (unusual because one doesn't often see a brown suit, it is not dark and staid, but rather, if you can imagine it, bright brown, and it looks good), seems unperturbed by what I experience as utter chaos.

When we finally get into his office (that he is called out three times while he is in there with us merely adds to the sense of general disorder), he is very engaging, smart, open, trusting our intelligence and our ability to make decisions. Looking at an MRI of my spine, he feels that physical therapy will do better than surgery (surgery, trust me, is not an option that I would even contemplate), especially given the complexity and generality of my geriatric spinal deterioration (he says it nicer than that, but we all know: aging is a bitch). So he has me go to physical therapy a few times a week for a few months. My therapist is a very engaging, attractive young woman, vainly trying to keep her boyfriend problems private. I like going because she does not insist on my doing those exercises I hate (eg. she does not easily understand my boredom on the stationary bicycle after just about twenty seconds, but she is willing to accept it) and she is very tolerant of my finally admitting that I do no exercises between appointments. And best of all, after a while, it does work, and the pain is gone.

One problem though. Richard sends me to an orthopedist for the pain in my wrist. The orthopedist is not sure that a cortisone shot will work because an X-ray of my wrist shows that arthritic and perhaps other changes have caused a space between bones that makes for a generally unstable situation there. He does give me the shot though (not an event for sissies, I must caution you), and to everyone's delight and my surprise, the pain goes away. A couple of months later, in physical therapy one day, the therapist, attempting to correct a problem I'm having with my shoulder, pulls my hand and the wrist pain is back. The pain is a familiar one to me, so I can tolerate it; I reassure the therapist that really it's no big deal and accept the fact that henceforth I have a very sore wrist. One learns to accommodate.

Although the very acute pain—the added pain from the Pompeii fall—gradually diminishes almost completely with the physical therapy (or would time alone have done it?), this thing with my calves seems to be getting worse. I used to describe it to Richard as, "It feels like nausea in my legs," because it didn't ache, it was just a mild unpleasantness that I was always aware of. But now, if I walk only two blocks my calves feel heavy, hot, and they do indeed hurt. If there is an incline of any sort, the pain in my legs starts right away. It's hard enough to function when your legs start to cry so easily, but in addition I am married to a woman who walks a lot—not only does she hike Sierra trails, she walks downtown, she walks everywhere. To accommodate, because she is very good to me, I accompany her on several walking trips (like the one I just mentioned, in Sicily), where she enjoys the walking and I enjoy the destination. I need to maintain some equilibrium in the marriage: she goes to movies for me, I walk for her—so I need to fix this leg problem. Richard refers me to a different vascular surgeon, this time, at my suggestion, at the medical school.

We call for an appointment and go to the specified floor in the medical center outpatient building. We follow the signs to *Vascular Surgery*, but where those signs lead finally is designated something else, the signage for *Vascular Surgery* having suddenly completely disappeared. We nonetheless approach a receptionist, tell her what we are looking for, she tells us to have a seat, that she will contact the appropriate person. We sit down in the waiting area, the point where two perpendicular corridors meet, the rows of seats at a forty-five degree angle to each corridor, the design choice arising, I expect, from not knowing which corridor to favor with parallel placement of chairs. Because of this design for the seating, because there is a large structural pillar in the middle of the seating area which blocks vision, the result is constant and considerable upper torso movement, back and forth, side to side, by seated patients who want to make sure that they are not forgotten by those in charge; timed more deliberately, it could be a Busby Berkeley number.

After a few minutes, the appropriate person comes out of an office to one side of the receptionist's desk (I guess it's like my father using space in a Kosher butcher shop Thursdays and Fridays to sell chickens; *Vascular Surgery* apparently shares somebody else's space and sells their chickens, as it were, Mondays). She has us fill out forms, takes us to an examining room, where we await The Man.

He turns out to be a rather mild man, who would be chosen in any casting call for a doctor. He looks the part perfectly: his doctor-ness is platonic, with his good looks, prematurely white hair, smooth skin on his sculpted face. He is accompanied (when introduced, the relationship is never clarified), every time we get together, by a tall, somewhat heavy-set younger man, (like Jack Carson in *Mildred Pierce*) whose large, round face looks boneless, he seems very smug, at best patronizing, arrogant, extremely clean, with very smooth, seemingly hairless skin. It looks like this is going to become good doc, bad doc! Pulses are groped for at my groin, thigh, ankle, foot,—by both hands of both people, on both sides of me—but faces are impassive and God knows what they learn, because no words are spoken to me. They're invading very personal space, getting pretty damn intimate with my body, but not a word to me about what they find, except later, when the groping is over, to say that my pain very likely reflects a condition called *intermittent claudication* and that it is most probably a result of my heavy smoking, even though I stopped smoking fifteen years before—wouldn't you know it! As my mother would have said, "My luck!"—the blood vessels do not dilate back to where they were before smoking constricted them.

Let me tell you a little about this condition. Intermittent claudication (I don't know what is intermittent in this situation; maybe it's because one walks only intermittently) is the name of the situation where there is insufficient blood flow to the legs, and therefore insufficient oxygen to the muscles, making walking very painful. Like so many other problems in life, the risk factors are smoking, genetics, high cholesterol, diabetes, obesity, and high blood pressure. Since I don't have high cholesterol, diabetes, obesity, and/or high blood pressure, what's left in my case is only smoking (about a pack and a half a day for forty one years) and genetics (my mother's toes having been amputated was a result of gangrene, because blood wasn't getting down there—but then too she was a heavy smoker).

They tell both Diana and me to start taking baby aspirins every night, immediately (my urologist doesn't tell me which kind of radiation I ought to choose for the prostate cancer, but these guys, we've barely been introduced and they are telling not only me, but also Diana, how to live;

how does she come under their rubric anyway; she's there to keep me company and get information, so their telling her to do aspirin is like you go to the movies and at the end Brandon de Wilde is shouting *your* name and asking *you* to come back) since that reduces the likelihood of heart attacks and they say it so urgently that I feel I ought to start it right then in their office.

This encounter brings to mind another unsolicited medical intervention, a situation involving my brother. He's at a social gathering, in short sleeves. A man comes up to him, introduces himself by name and as a dermatologist, and tells him that he's concerned about something on my brother's arm and that he ought to make an appointment to come into his office to have it removed and biopsied (quite a marketing technique: go to parties and enlarge your patient base). Might I suggest an analogy? Imagine I am at a party, I sidle up to somebody, and say that his/her behavior at the event seems iffy to me and that he/she ought to call for an appointment to see me for psychotherapy. Do I go too far?

At any rate, the vascular people refer me for some kind of test where blood pressure cuffs are placed the length of both legs and arterial pressures are compared and sonograms of the arteries are done.

Following the test, there's a second visit to the dyad and this time the good guy explains what he thinks is going on, what the tests confirm, what the possibilities are, but says that, though he doesn't think it will work, the conservative first approach is that I am to walk twelve blocks a day for ten weeks, that sometimes, actually only rarely, despite narrowed or closed abdominal and femoral arteries, that kind of exercise works. It's not that I'm to build up to twelve a day; it's at twelve that I am to start. So, get this: even though the pain makes walking two blocks very difficult—it really hurts a lot—and even though he admits that there is almost no likelihood that it will work, I'm supposed to do twelve blocks a day! Is this a step toward my beatification or simply an S&M strategy on his part?

I try. I cheat a little because the discomfort is unbearable, but, for the most part, I suffer through it, tears in my eyes—if anything, my hunch is that it's the journey toward martyrdom that is going to make it work—but, after the ten weeks, the amount of pain and the number of blocks I can walk before the pain starts do not change; that is to say, just as predicted, the agonizing walking I've been doing has been, alas, to no avail.

So we go back for a third visit. This time they want me to have an MRA from my abdomen down (and he says MRA with an aggressive accent on the A to make sure, I think, that I don't question whether he meant an MRI. MRA, by the way, stands for Magnetic Resonance Angiography. It is a kind of MRI—in MRI, the I stands for _imaging_—but in an MRA, instead of other tissue, it is the arteries that are exposed and delineated) in order to confirm the problem with the abdominal and femoral arteries. (Actually, how much confirmation do we need? Isn't there enough confirming evidence by now? Does he get a cut of the cost of these tests?) His office arranges an appointment and a clerk gives me a form that says I have an appointment several days thence at 1:00PM and that I am not to eat after midnight the night before. The scheduled day, I get to Radiology at about 12:50, very hungry, and in my shirt pocket is a Hershey bar with which to break the fast—I'm sure that I will not be able to wait to get to the cafeteria afterwards—and I sign in with the clerk.

At 1:30 (i.e. half an hour after the appointment time), dizzy with hunger, I return to the desk and ask why I've not been called, and the clerk says that my appointment is at 2:00. I show her my referral papers on which 1:00PM is very clearly written, she shows me her book in which there is no mistake that I am in the 2:00PM slot. Rather than risk what she no doubt fears will be a physical assault (imagine the angry vibes I'm giving off), she calls a young man out of somewhere, he apologizes for the discrepancy in appointment time, saying that it is impossible to know at which end the error was made, I say that the source of the error really doesn't matter to me at this point. He says that he will get to me as quickly as possible, even though they are a bit behind today. I say that I hope so, since I am very hungry, he suggests I get something to eat in the cafeteria, I show him my referral forms where it very clearly states that I am to have no food after midnight the night before, and he says that this prohibition is surely an error, that there is no reason that my stomach need be empty. It's clear to me who is making the mistakes now—and it ain't Radiology. I return to my seat, take the now vastly melted Hershey bar from my pocket, peel as much of the paper from the soft mess as I can, essentially lick up the candy, trying to avoid dripping and to make sure that I look like I don't care what the other waiting people think.

At the next appointment, the vascular surgeon says that the MRA supports his view about my abdominal and femoral arteries. Also, he says that it shows that my kidney problems (he comments on kidney problems because my blood tests for years now have shown high creatinine levels; when creatinine levels are high, one assumes that there are kidney problems) are not due to a decreased blood supply to the kidney (I could have told him that. I could have told him that my "kidney problems" are due to my having only one kidney and my being old!) Here's the deal about

Creatinine. Creatinine is a protein released by muscle into the blood. The kidney filters waste products out of blood, and creatinine is a waste product. If kidneys are impaired, the creatinine level in the blood rises because it is being filtered out less efficiently, more slowly, so there is more in the blood. A normal level of creatinine is 1.0 (normal range is .8 to 1.4 or thereabouts, depending on the institution giving out the numbers). My creatinine level has ranged between 1.6 and 2.3, at least since I started in the Gleevec triala and have been given the results of every blood test. This means (very grossly) that my kidney is functioning at about 50 % of what a person with two normal kidneys would be doing.

Again, he says that he wants to be conservative, so he puts me on a drug called Pletal which he says is a Japanese drug, sometimes helpful with intermittent claudication, though the mechanism is not known, and gives me an appointment for several weeks later—far enough away to give the drug a chance to work. His position again is that before arranging for angioplasty or bypasses, let's try more conservative approaches.

Conservative? Oh, yeah, sure! I spend the next few days sick to my stomach, short of breath, my heart pounding, and on the fourth day, after vomiting, I have to stay at home while Diana takes out-of-town friends on a sightseeing drive. I call the office, am told that one of the nurses will call me back, play a little phone tag, and finally get someone on the phone. I tell her my problem, she says that she will speak to the doctor, and will call me back: more phone tag and finally she reaches me and tells me that the doctor says that I should stop taking the Pletal; I ask for an appointment, she will have to get back to me, and there we go again with phone tag.

The basic question here is why I can't speak directly to the doctor. Why must there always be an intermediary whose presence at least doubles the amount of work in setting up each transaction? What does it mean about this fellow that he is unwilling to speak to patients on the phone? Finally I get an appointment (after many messages are left by each of us on a variety of phones, she gets me on my cell phone while I'm in front of a book-art gallery to which I've brought those out-of-town guests whom I mentioned before, we set up an appointment and I go in a few days later.

The vascular surgeon explains that my vascular situation is such that I can have angioplasty in the femoral artery in the right leg, but not in the left where the artery is too closed down to allow the insertion of a balloon, so a bypass will be necessary there. I want to do both procedures at the same time; he explains that it is important that the wound (that's the word he uses; sounds like a big deal, doesn't it?) from the angioplasty heal completely prior to an incision close-by for the by-pass, so we'll do one, then schedule the other.

He also explains that there are two kinds of by-passes, and even though using a graft taken from a vein is a more complicated procedure, requiring more surgery (that is, you have first to remove a piece of vein and then to replace a section of artery with it) and thus more healing than a by-pass using synthetic materials, the venous one is better and that is what he is planning to do. (It stands to reason, doesn't it, that the complicated procedure, the one that will require more recovery time, is his choice. I don't get it.) He says that he is troubled by the high creatinine in my blood tests and would like me to see a kidney specialist before the angioplasty; that his office will contact me when they've been able to schedule the angioploasty; that I will have to come in the day before the procedure is scheduled, at noon, in order to take some medicine and also be hydrated, both of these in order to minimize damage to my one kidney.

I arrange to see a nephrologist (do you too find this title a little too close to *necrologist*?), a kidney specialist (imagine the number of rather arcane specialists I now have in my rolodex!). Dr. Santiesteban is a welcoming, warm man, with one earring and a carelessly knotted Versace tie, who says that my high creatinine is reasonable and to be expected because, in people over 55, when a kidney is removed, the remaining one does not take over the function of the one that's been removed. (Yes. he did say, "The remaining one does not take over the function of the one that's been removed!!!!" Now wait a minute! Does this mean that everyone has been lying to me up to now, or do these doctors, knowledgeable in their own specialties, simply not know much about kidneys? Well if they don't know for sure, why are they so quick to offer me such definite reassurance that turns out to be bogus?)

He estimates that my kidney function is thirty to forty percent of what it should be. (Frightening! What happens to those functions that my one kidney is not able to accomplish? It would stand to reason that it's not only creatinine that's not being filtered out of my blood! How much gunk can my blood retain?) And then, like a lightning bolt it hits me: does this mean also that I'm making only thirty to forty percent of the erythropoietin I should have? And can that explain some of what I've thought were side effects of Gleevec? His answer to each is a very emphatic *yes*. I'm not really sure why, but this knowledge is very reassuring to me. I suppose that the reassurance

125

comes from the fact that there is finally an explanation for problems that I'm having. This, despite my knowledge now that my blood is filling up with waste products and my question of how long that can go on. I am also dismayed that no one has put these particular two and two together before

Sometimes, in bed at night, just before sleeping, I allow myself to reckon with the enormity of the consequences of my nephrectomy: I can no longer enter any medical encounter with trust, because I have been deceived and/ or misinformed repeatedly about issues relating to my kidneys; I worry, with good reason especially considering my age, that my creatinine will rise further, indicating that my remaining kidney is inadequate; I put up with several years of very serious discomfort and other problems relating to the inadequate production of erythropoietin. I allow these ruminations only in darkness, as though the light of day will keep these thoughts spiraling into obsessions and rage.

So it's time for me to be admitted to the hospital for the angioplasty. I have some awareness of how things work in hospitals and of the ample opportunity that problems there afford for power trips, I have developed some ability to predict what is going to raise hackles, and yet I foolishly call radiology (the department that is responsible for the procedure I'm being admitted for and is to take place the following day: the angioplasty), speak to a nurse, and ask her, as though I need her permission, as though everybody in the world comes to things exactly on time, as if there is going to be no wait when I arrive, if she thinks there will be any problem if I come in to be admitted at 2:00PM instead of at noon (the tai chi class that Diana has persuaded me into a while back—that's a whole other story—having completed an entire year, is having a little graduation party at 11:30).

She pulls an attitude (she is now Louise Fletcher in *One Flew Over the Cuckoo's Nest)*, says that she, of course, can't tell me what to do (then, exactly what does she think she's doing?), but that if they said I should be there at noon, they didn't mean 2:00. (It's like I'm in second grade again! And keep in mind that I'm being admitted at noon for a procedure that is to take place the following morning.) I acknowledge that that's very likely true, but that sometimes admissions procedures take longer, sometimes the people who are supposed to do the tasks for which I'm being admitted a day early don't arrive so quickly, and if I'm in at 2:00, there are still eight or nine hours to do the few necessary tasks, and we have all night to hydrate, what is the problem! I'm trying to be logical, to convince her, not to argue with her, but as I talk I feel her becoming more rigid and her attitude sharpens; she tries to make me feel like a delinquent, like I'm trying to get away with something, that I'm trying to put something over on the medical establishment!

Finally, sanity prevails for me (that is, I stop the conversation before I blow up); I thank her and I get off the phone. I decide to do what I should have done to begin with, compromise somewhat, this time without telling anyone, and the next day, I go to the party for a short while, eat a little lunch there, leave, accompanied by the good wishes of my tai-chi partners, and then arrive at hospital admissions a little before 1:00PM.

After a forty minute wait in the admissions office (yes indeed, forty minutes!), the clerk calls me over, looks at my papers, and wants to send me up to radiology because that's what's on the form the vascular people have given me. (Remember my MRA referral slip? These referrers are batting 1000) It is clear to me that the clerk's understanding of the referral is very different from what I'm really there for and from what had been planned by the vascular people. These vascular people simply do not make things very clear on their referrals! I explain that, "No, actually I'm supposed to be sent to an in-patient unit and tomorrow a procedure will be done in Radiology," and finally after much telephoning, interviewing, head scratching, and chewing on pencils by the clerical people, I'm sent to the tenth floor, and given a bed.

As the day goes on, the tasks that need to get done (those that the radiology nurse on the phone was worried that I wouldn't have time for) get done in a rather leisurely manner—just as I would have predicted, nobody seems to be in any particular rush. I am told that my hemoglobin is *very* low and that, in the evening, they will be giving me a couple of units of blood, so that I will not be anemic during the procedure which is scheduled for early morning. They tell me this in the most matter-of-fact, breezy manner, as though everyone knows that on Thursdays one has transfusions.

You might notice that what I don't hear is any curiosity about the source of the anemia; I mean, true, I've been marginally anemic since all this started, but not anywhere near needing transfusions, so you'd think that those who notice this new level of anemia might wonder about its source. I am in a hospital, after all, they can probably get me at any hour for whatever tests that might be useful, all they have to do is whistle. But, no—correcting this problem, whatever it is, with a transfusion seems to be enough for these folks. So I get the blood and feel better than I've felt perhaps in years! I see my surgeon's younger and heavier shadow—let's call him *Doctor B*—he tells me a little about what's going to happen, and says that I will probably be spending the next night too in the hospital, since we have to be concerned about my kidney and be vigilant about what goes on with it.

My roommate, a genial, articulate middle-aged man, with hints of the picaresque and, judging by his verbal reactions to newscasters on TV, politics similar to mine, provides just the right amount of company. He talks with considerable charm and openness about his background and about his family in a way that is by no means intrusive and he also expresses interest in my experience. He is in the hospital because of chest pains, although he looks to me to be in very good shape. There is no way I can fail to hear, despite the curtain drawn around his bed, the conversations he has with doctors, who explain to him that, after a few more tests, they will surely be recommending heart surgery and to whom he expresses his willingness to go by their recommendation.

When they leave he confides that he is made extremely anxious by the prospect of the surgery and, as much as possible for a layman and a shrink, I offer reassurance. Then a priest comes in and, in their ensuing conversation, we learn (the priest, who, like the doctors, has drawn the curtain around my roommate's bed) that he has not taken communion in many years and the priest offers him that and apparently other rituals, to ensure salvation, just in case. I know that that's a lot better reassurance than I can offer. I've done a lot of reading and I've seen my Graham Green movies.

The next morning my procedure is done early, without incident. Let me describe the procedure. I'm lying on a table. The radiologist is sitting by my side at my hip. She inserts a needle in the left side of my groin (remember the leg they're doing is the right one) and is able to inject a dye into the arteries on both legs in order to have pictures of both sets of blood vessels, and through that same incision to insert a balloon into the artery on the right side in order to dilate it (the artery) so that the blood flow will improve.

The radiologist who does this procedure is a very quiet woman, hair pulled back, no make-up, and gives the impression that she cherishes her drabness (in the movies, she would be the person who, close to the last scene, out of love for the hero, lets her hair down, takes off her glasses, the lighting changes, as does her make-up—and she has become BEAUTIFUL; it's not always out of love, sometimes—like Dorothy Malone in *The Big Sleep*—it can be just good old lust.).

She seems reluctant to communicate with me at all, as though any connection with the person with whom she is dealing (me!), beyond the line that she is inserting into my groin and the image on the monitor, would be an anathema to her; she does, of course, introduce herself—we are civilized!—but then, in response to a question of mine before she starts the procedure, she says quietly, directly, and with no humor, that during the procedure she does not want to be distracted by questions from me (her attitude communicates that I've already been a bad boy to raise any question, to talk at all), and then, even when the procedure is finished, she says nothing at all to me. Well, maybe "Goodbye."

In addition to my disappointment at her social reticence, it is a problem for me that during the procedure I am lying flat on the bed and not allowed to raise my head, with the result that I am not even able to watch any of the procedure on the monitor; not being able to watch means that even a pretext of control is denied me. It's amusing that I have to keep my mouth shut, because during the procedure, perhaps ten feet away from us, staff is coming in and out of an office, having conversations, discussing schedules. The traffic and the ruckus are very distracting to me, but I guess not to her.

The radiologist does nod at me when she comes into the recovery area to instruct a young resident or medical student (whatever! No one identifies these hierarchical statuses) about how to put pressure on the small incision (this wound that the vascular surgeon was so worried about and that has to heal for a while before the by-pass can be done is like a pin prick!) for about a half hour, in order that clots not develop and screw up the newly opened arterial pathway. She leaves and the resident stands there, pressing his fingers into the left side of my groin for the entire half hour, checking the clock frequently. I try to make jokes about this somewhat awkward situation, but he clearly is not willing to see any humor in what he has been told to do, however strange it might be. My jokes fall flat, he responds to any comments I make with as few words as possible, I don't want to torment him, so we pass the time awkwardly, mostly in silence; but, it is true, no clots develop later to cause problems.

With that over, I'm brought back to my floor. I'm surprised that Diana is not there waiting for me, because that's what she would usually have done. She shows up a little later, looking a bit flummoxed, and here's the story: she comes to the floor earlier and asks where my procedure is taking place; the nurse she speaks with at the nursing station asks her what the procedure was to have been (could this nurse be unaware perhaps that there are files and computers replete with information about me and what I am in the hospital for?). Diana says that it is an angioplasty, so the nurse sends her upstairs where cardiac angioplasties are done, instead of downstairs to Radiology where my thigh is being dealt with. Nobody upstairs knows who I am (they too apparently don't know about nor have access to computers, or at least in their heads it's more efficient that she schlepp all over the hospital searching for me, than that they spend a minute at the computer), so it's a bad scene for her all around; Diana comes back to my floor, not knowing what to expect, and there I am.

Mid-afternoon, the wonderful, informative, solicitous nurse—a mensch, in other words: a nurse who functions the way you expect and want nurses to function—who is assigned to me, tells me that he's overheard the doctors (who these doctors are is always a mystery, since I don't apparently have access to them—it's not the radiologist, she doesn't talk to me, it's not my main vascular guy, he doesn't even show up, it must be Doctor B; engaging me in a planning process about myself seems to be a primary taboo in my hospital situation) saying that I will probably be leaving the hospital late in the afternoon. Later, when Doctor B comes around, I ask about what time I might be discharged. He says, as though I'm a misbehaving five year old or, even worse perhaps, a doddering old man, verging on senility, "Don't you remember what I told you last evening, that you will not be discharged until tomorrow?" What I don't say is "What I remember most is that you are an arrogant, smug, condescending prick;" instead I merely say, "Of course."

I ask why the radiologist has not put in a stent, a mesh tube that prevents the artery from narrowing down again (because the radiologist didn't tell me she hadn't—she didn't tell me anything!—I didn't learn that she hadn't put one in until after she had left the scene, so I was not able to ask her; I would have expected, on the basis of what had been explained to me before the surgery, that a stent would be used to make sure that the artery stays open over time) and he says, "She didn't have to," as though the last thing someone in my situation needs is information.

It's a curious thing that too often, when doctors give answers like this, I (and, I expect, most of the rest of the population) sometimes don't pursue more information. I think there are several reasons. The definiteness of their statements, even though they may mean nothing, takes me by surprise, I suppose that I don't recognize the nonsense immediately, and I don't recoup in time to ask further. It is also very seductive to be mindless, to let them do the thinking; they are the pros, so you cede your critical faculties and simply accept what they say and by the time you realize what has happened, it's too late to go back. In addition, I am afraid that pushing my question is going to sound hostile and I don't want people with responsibility for my arteries (or any other part of my body) to become defensive or feel hostile toward me in return. So, at times my position, in a sense, demands that I opt instead for no information.

My nurse, the mensch referred to above, was assigned to me for the day I came into the hospital and the day of the procedure. The following day, the day on which I am to be discharged at about 1:00 PM, a different nurse is assigned to me, even though the mensch guy is also on duty that day. Score one for continuity of care! I realize that there may be many reasons for the switch: I need less or, more likely, no care this third day—but if that's the case, why assign me any nurse? Or that the mensch can't stand me is, of course, a possibility. Or, for example, it just worked out that way—whatever. But one would think that there might be a short conversation with me early in the day, at least to acknowledge that a switch is taking place and maybe even to tell me why.

I am discharged this anticipated third day, with a prescription for Plavix (a drug which does something to make platelets less able to clot, in order to ensure smooth blood flow through the recently repaired artery; otherwise clots might screw everything up by creating a new barrier in the artery), my right leg no longer hurts, and I feel terrific for four more days after the transfusion and then I'm back to huffing and puffing and feeling that death is imminent. I go for a routine appointment with Charlie, tell him about the transfusion, tell him that I'm sapped, dizzy, and breathless again. We talk about my kidney and erythropoietin, and he tells me he can get rid of these symptoms by putting me on Procrit. (Remember, he and all the others were pooh-poohing the possibility of Procrit for me over the previous three or four years. Perhaps there has been a recent article in JAMA or in some hematology journal advocating Procrit for marginal anemia!). I am delighted, they give me a shot before I leave, I have the prescription filled when I get home, and now I know I'm in business. Four days later I'm feeling lousy again, and so it goes for the next four weeks: I feel good for four days after the weekly Procrit shot and then I feel lousy, short of breath, very tired for three days.

Then my follow-up visit with the vascular people—everything's the way it should be—and we're preparing for the by-pass one week later. My doctor and Dr. B and a resident I've never seen before get up to leave after just a couple of minutes of nothing conversation and I say, "Please! Just a minute. Could we talk about the anesthesia?" and they sit down again and tell me about the anesthesia, I tell them about my reluctance to be unconscious, my need (as you might have guessed from some of these stories) to feel a little control, to which he says that he doesn't want me talking and distracting him during surgery (he and the radiologist must have been in the same *How to Win Friends and Influence People* seminar); I promise, and he says that I can discuss the choices later with the anesthesiologist, and they get up to leave.

"No. No," say I. "Please. About how long will the recovery be and what will it be like?" They sit down and talk about what I may expect, and then get up again to leave. Their getting up and sitting down by now has the feel of a Marx Brothers movie. "Wait a sec," I say. They laugh and again sit down, and I ask: "In what way is the vein graft better than the synthetic one?"

Immediately, the atmosphere becomes uncomfortable. The air now is suddenly thick with tension. Dr. B looks at his colleagues (seemingly in disbelief) and then somewhat sternly at me, and my doctor says, "In five years, the probability is 15% that the vein graft will do better than one using synthetic material. Now, this study was done without using a particular medication (I am not sure, but I think it is Plavix), but if that medication is used, I would judge that there is no difference." "Then why," I ask, "would anyone choose the vein over the synthetic? It seems that nothing is to be gained over the synthetic one and it is a more difficult undertaking and I am an old man. I want the synthetic one." "That's reasonable," he says and they leave. Well, if it's so goddamn reasonable now, why were they insisting on this tortuous vein thing until this very moment? There seems to be something here that doesn't quite make sense, unless, of course, there is a resident who needs some experience grafting veins! Well, then tell me that and let me make a choice; at least things won't sound so arbitrary and foolish!

I am told to stop the Plavix one week before the surgery. I suppose, but am not sure, that I am to continue with the aspirin, but that doesn't quite make sense to me. They want bleeding to be controllable during surgery and to stop after surgery and that's why I am to stop the Plavix. I'm not sure what role aspirin plays in this bleeding thing, but I think it does play one; still nobody has mentioned aspirin to me now and they did tell me about Plavix. So I call to ask about the aspirin and it's the same situation as before. I finally am able to get a nurse, who will call me back after she's spoken with the doctor. She calls later to say that I should stay on the aspirin. Three phone calls, two hours! And still no explanation.

I show up a week later, two days before the surgery is scheduled, for the pre-op stuff, and a very pleasant, considerate, thoughtful, somewhat self-effacing young resident (at first I'm afraid that he'll never make it in this field; but then, very quickly, I realize that it's still very early in his career—there will be plenty of opportunity for him to develop the apparently necessary arrogance, during the considerable mentoring yet to take place), whom I've not met before, examines me, apologizing repeatedly for the broom-closet or storage room look of the area and he says that he has some papers for me to sign.

One of them gives permission for them to do a venous graft. Now, I don't believe (despite my experience with the kidney and my resulting paranoia) that they slipped that in on purpose and will do that kind of surgery if I sign it, but it surely is something to ponder! Why wouldn't they have specified carefully the surgery that we'd decided on—especially since I've made such a point of it? If they had thought about it, would they really expect me to be signing this? I tell the resident to change it, he does, and before I am ready to leave, I ask him for a copy of my blood work. He returns with the printout and points out that my hemoglobin and hematocrit are very low indeed; this after five weeks on Procrit!

So I get home fast and e-mail Charlie—never forget about Charlie, my leukemia guy and hero—about the situation. He has become my shaman. He must have sensed desperation in my email, because he calls me at home immediately and has me come in. (Notice: he calls me. He doesn't have a secretary call and give me a message. I once faxed him a note, asking for some information for an aunt of mine just diagnosed with a different kind of leukemia; he called me immediately to talk about it.) He is baffled and doesn't mind my seeing that! My newly acquired anemia, he feels strongly, cannot be a function of my leukemia and he outlines the reasons for that.

He thinks that I must be bleeding somewhere, but I cannot help him with that: I've seen no blood. He repeatedly asks me what has been different lately; I can think of nothing. Any change in medication?—and there it is: I've added over the last several months aspirin, Pletal, and Plavix. I tell him that I stopped the Plavix a week ago in preparation for the surgery and would stop the aspirins as of this day. He calls the vascular surgeon who cancels the surgery, because, after a by-pass with a synthetic, I would have to be on aspirin and Plavix, and until we are sure whether they are or are not the cause of my probable bleeding, no surgery.

I find this very disturbing: the vascular guy has put me on these drugs, my blood counts are available to him in my records on the computer, he'd noticed that I was anemic at the time of the angioplasty—it was, after all, his people who ordered the blood transfusion the night before that procedure—my radical nephrectomy is certainly in my records, and after "Hello", it's the first thing I mention to doctors who are new to me, shouldn't he have put two and two together? Why does it have to be Charlie, who gets into the picture now only because I've appealed to him, and not these vascular people, who ends up putting together the relationship between the drugs and the anemia?

Charlie has me come in for a couple of units of blood the following day. Every couple of weeks a transfusion? Isn't there a limit? As days pass though, now off aspirin and Plavix, I notice that the effects of this transfusion are lasting longer than a week, instead of what had been the usual four days. In addition, it is taking a lot further than two blocks for my left leg to start hurting. Could it be that more oxygen is getting to the muscle as a result of the transfusion of blood more oxygenated than mine and, now that it is being prescribed again, the Procrit? Wow! All those tests, the MRAs, the sonograms—could they have been set aside for a while if someone had taken my very frequent blood tests more seriously.

Here's my take on what's happened now: instead of increasing the flow of somewhat anemic blood through the arteries to my legs and thus giving the muscles a bit more oxygen, which is what the angioplasty did and what the by-pass would do, getting on Procrit and off Plavix has increased the amount of red cells in the blood that my capillaries are bringing to my legs and, in that way, we have enriched the oxygen flow to the muscles. I'm not sure about vascular physiology; what I do know is that my walking situation these days seems just about normal to me. The fact is that on a recent trip to Italy, I managed, without pain, to walk two, three, four miles a day. Nobody seems to have thought of increasing my red cells before! It would seem to me that that approach (this one now accidentally taken) is more conservative and certainly more economical in every way than an angioplasty and a bypass. I am aware that I still have some serious vascular problems, but I can take my time, without the pressure of pain, to decide how and when I want to deal with them.

I am perplexed. I am relatively intelligent and thoughtful; as you remember I had worked in a hospital many years, I pretty much know the system and am generally wary, all of which characterizes me as a sophisticated consumer of medical services, and yet all this befalls me. If I am beset by these problems, what happens to people less sophisticated than I am—how do they maneuver through a system that I—good old knowledgeable, experienced me—have such terrible trouble with. Maybe these other people never expect humane, empathic treatment. Maybe they don't notice. Maybe they don't mind being treated like a leg, or a kidney, or whatever—but how can any of that be true? What I think personally is that they must quietly die.

What I really seem to need now is someone to organize all my medical findings, to make sense of all these things across specialties—what we used to call a case manager. We all do! Richard, my primary physician—remember him from the first pages and a few pop-ins here and there?—can't even begin to carry on with that function, because, first of all, not part of the University system, he doesn't even get most of findings. No matter how I implore the clerks wherever I find myself medically, they don't always send him the stuff. And now, in this saga of mine, with referrals being made by specialists to other specialists, Richard is completely out of the loop. And, I hate to talk about money, but there is, of course, also the almost certainty that Medicare won't allow billing for that kind of activity and I want Richard to make a good living. Charlie can't do case management; he does have the heart and the heroism, but he did choose, after all, to be in a specialty, in academic medicine, in the oncology business, and has a lot to keep him busy there.

While we're on the subject of medical records let me tell you a little story. Diana had a mammogram and they wanted to compare the film with previous mammograms she'd had. There were two medical centers involved, so she got on the phone with each of them and after a number of calls to medical records and x-ray libraries at each, she discovered that nobody knew where the films might be and she was cautioned by several people to keep possession of these films from now on herself, that otherwise this sort of thing is likely to happen again. And then, we both remembered, to our excruciating embarrassment that, after the last mammogram, she had brought home all her mammogram films and that they were in a closet here at home. We ourselves, then, it turns out, are not too dependable as our own medical managers.

Despite this, it seems that I have to become my own organizer, in effect, my own primary physician. I really don't know enough to play that role well and sometimes, when decisions have to be made, I am, as you no doubt remember, anesthetized. But when I'm awake, I do have logic, intelligence, a memory for what happened yesterday, I do care dearly about consequences to my life, and I have some breadth of interest—qualities that some of my practitioners with more specific medical knowledge have lacked. But keep in mind what happened with Diana's mammogram records that we were trying to take charge of;

we are not as well organized as we'd want and our memory seems to have holes. But if I don't do it, nobody is going to do it, and, despite all the technology and good intentions, I will be adrift, as I fear we all are. It is not managed care that is the danger here; the danger is more that there is no manager of the care we get.

One more thing I'd like you to know. Every year, you might remember, in the spring, I have a CT scan, both to make sure that my renal cell carcinoma has not popped up somewhere and, I guess, also to remind me annually that I am not yet to consider myself free of a worrisome problem. The CT scans have taken place through a variety of my moods and physical states; it would have been hard to predict, when we started them, what my situation would be in the spring of each subsequent year. Once, early in my Gleevec career, when I was taking the pills two hours after breakfast, thus on an empty stomach, while changing into a hospital gown in the locker room, I and of course the CT scan personnel were lucky that I found a wastebasket for me to vomit into! That kind of inconvenience is in the past; nowadays it is a joy, every year, to read the report indicating negative results.

VIII

In which attempts to discover if there is internal bleeding and, if so, its source, create more frustrations, all of which I try to master.

The events that arise here are not the life-death variety; their consequences have more to do with anxiety than with physical pain and disability. Yet I think this story is especially relevant, because, with its own particular flavor, it picks up, captures, and reflects many of the threads, the issues, the problems that I've been dealing with until now. The point is that even in less serious arenas, those which don't involve the possibility of dire results, the same kinds of issues—the irrational rigidity of the system, the thoughtlessness, the dehumanization, that everything revolves around the procedure, the routine, and the convenience of the practitioner rather than the patient—gnaw. So here goes.

It has been decided that an endoscopy and a colonoscopy will tell us more specifically where the source of the bleeding that's causing the anemia might be, (assuming that it is indeed bleeding that is causing the anemia), so we call the gastroenterologist to schedule an appointment. The phone rings four times and then there's a message indicating that this is the practice of the gastroenterologist (by name) and the nurse practitioner (also by name), and one is advised which number to press if one is a patient. Despite my tendency to obsess, I quickly decide that even though they have not yet met me and I am therefore not yet their patient, *patient* is the closest category to my status, i.e., I don't want to be part of the gastric bypass surgery program (call a different number), I am not an emergency (hang up and dial 911), and I am not a physician (press one), so I press two.

Does it really make sense to have the same kind of relationship with our doctors that we have with our phone company? Surely I know the reasons that this kind of phone tree gets to be used. That it saves both kinds of enterprises money and time, however, is beside the point, since the bases of these two kinds of encounters are vastly different. Being instructed by a recorded voice puts me off quite a bit even when my needs are impersonal. But when I need a doctor, the emotional, personal needs involved make it imperative to talk to a real person. The very fact that I am trying to make an appointment with a physician would indicate that I am concerned, nervous about something, right? The impersonality of a recorded voice certainly does not alleviate my anxiety; the frustration in not making direct contact certainly exacerbates the anxiety.

This issue calls up those outpatient settings, like labs, where you are asked to take a number when you come in and wait until your number is called, before you get the service you are there for. I am not comfortable with those numbers even in a bakery or at the DMV, let alone in a medical setting, but I don't set policy. Still in other medical settings you are expected to stand in line; there is often a yellow stripe painted on the floor, and a rather inconspicuous sign saying, "Please stand behind the line until you are called"; because the sign is inconspicuous, one might pass the stripe by accident and then be reprimanded for having stepped over the stripe and be told to stand behind it, even though there is nobody else waiting. Being *called* often means that the clerk yells out, "Next," or something equally unpleasant. Standing in line and taking a number are the humiliating ways that marginalized people get their marginalization reinforced, for example, in welfare offices. It's the last thing people concerned about their health need.

Another set-up is the one where you're asked to sign in and wait until your name is called, frequently mispronounced, often merely spelled out, almost always lacking a Mr. or Ms—a method, from most points of view, neither successful, nor pleasant: many people are private and don't want their names yelled out in public, and calling people simply by their last name cuts off a big hunk of dignity, it diminishes the person. There are those who feel dehumanized by a number and there are those who want no one to hear their names. I, of course, am willing to hear my name called, rather than suffer the bakery model; but I do know that there are others who will put up with what I view as not human, rather than risk their name being called out in public. Well, which are we to support: paranoia or humanism? For me the preference will always be that I be seen as a person, by a person whom I recognize as human. But surely there are other options, with different methods of staffing, so that the whole thing can be designed to be done more personally.

And while we're on the subject of outpatient settings, how about those offices in which, when you enter for the first time, you are somewhat at a loss because there is no employee to talk with, no one to whom you can announce your arrival? There might be other patients sitting around, but they don't care about your arrival, and you would feel a little dumb asking them what the procedure is; they apparently figured it out and you want to seem a little cool, a little sophisticated to them. There is often a sliding, translucent glass panel, and you know that the clerical staff is on the other side of it, (you do hear voices and clerical sounds), but what are you supposed to do to make sure that they know you've arrived. The choices are: knock on the window, slide it open, or do nothing—i.e., wait them out; they have surely heard the door open, let it be their problem. Your mother is not around to tell you what to do, and there is no sign with instructions. No matter what you choose, you will know immediately that what you decided is the wrong way to do it.

Sorry for the digressions, but I did warn you a long time ago. Anyway, finally, after the right buttons have been pressed, a real woman answers. I tell her my situation and she tells me that there is no appointment available on Monday (this is Friday and I have certainly not even hinted that I need an appointment on the next business day), but that, nonetheless, she will squeeze me in. Why squeeze me in? I can wait a while. And if they are going to squeeze me in, why mention that there are no openings? Why do I have to know that? Would they squeeze anybody in, or have they heard something about me? Am I supposed to feel indebted?

We get there early—we get everywhere early—and I give the clerk my name and insurance cards and she gives me a somewhat longer than usual, four page history and organ systems form; she asks me to sit down and fill it out. The waiting room is crowded, but there are two empty seats, not together; without our asking, there is some quick shifting of chairs so that Diana and I are able to sit together. I sit and start to fill out the form. I have an itch on my cheek,

I scratch it, and realize that I had some kind of little abrasion and have now broken the skin. I am bleeding.

I try to stop the bleeding by pressing Kleenex onto the source, but the bleeding does not stop. I go into the bathroom, at the other end of the hall from the gastroenterologist's office, partly to get away from the gaze of the others in the waiting room and partly to have water available (as though water will do something I need), I try using toilet paper, Kleenex, paper towels, each with a lot of pressure, and the bleeding does not decrease. I try folding up a small piece of Kleenex and, like when I cut myself shaving, putting it on the cut. The Kleenex is saturated with blood before I remove my finger. I'm there to find out why I'm anemic, where I'm bleeding from, and here I am, bleeding from a new place uncontrollably!

I grab a fistful of Kleenex and paper towels and leave the bathroom, since I'm having no luck there—the presence of water hasn't helped. I'm trying very hard to be cool; panic in a doctor's waiting room is not something I want to try out. I sit there, filling out the form and then reading, one hand pressing whatever kind of absorbent paper I've chosen for that moment onto my cheek.

I know that some of the elderly people in the waiting area—they are all elderly people—are feeling sorry for me, thinking that my lack of clotting is the result of some cancer treatment reducing platelets (one woman does acknowledge her sympathy to my wife while I'm in the bathroom). As you might have guessed, I cannot stand their feeling sorry for me. And I cannot stand being seen as unable to control this particular function of mine: bleeding. On the other hand, I'm almost not worried about why this is happening, because, if our hunch is right, having stopped the Plavix only four days before and still on aspirin, I'm still, temporarily a bleeder, or at least not an efficient blood clotter. As the clock ticks away, however, I do start to worry about how much blood I can afford to lose.

After forty-five minutes (I'm thinking "We'll squeeze you in" is a ploy this office uses with everyone who presses the number two: by setting things up like they're doing you a favor, they are going to minimize the likelihood of patients complaining about the wait, of rebellions starting in the waiting room), the nurse practitioner calls us into an office and, before we sit down, comments about my bleeding ("Gee, you are really bleeding!" she says. "Gee, you are really perceptive!" I want to say, but don't.), which has continued to saturate whatever I've used to apply pressure to the source of the bleeding now for forty minutes. (How long till I run out of blood?) I smile and say (stiff-upper-lip fashion) that it will be fine, that I'm on top of it, but fortunately she sees that I'm not and insists on getting me a gauze pad and advises pressure (actually I want the gauze pad, but not the advice; what does she think I've been doing all this time? Doesn't she see me pressing?).

She then starts the very mechanical history interview; the idea of going down a list of organ systems again is excruciating to me (especially since, while bleeding, I've just filled out that form in the waiting room, giving all the information she's going to be asking for, making certain that I'm not getting any blood on the form; what do they do with these forms after they have been filled out anyway? Do they have you fill them out just to keep you busy as a second maneuver to reduce the likelihood of any disruption by those waiting so long? Are these forms then an anti-mutiny device?), so I interrupt as shyly and nicely as I am able (at least I'm trying to be nice!), and suggest that I can give her my relevant history myself, without prompts from her list, that I can do it chronologically, articulately and clearly, (that is, we can have a human encounter) if she doesn't mind. She says that she doesn't mind, but actually she gives off the impression that she does; you can just tell. Nonetheless, we finish the history my way.

She leaves, and after a few minutes the bleeding stops. After a short while (during which no one appears at the door to inquire about the bleeding), she comes back to take us to a room where the doctor will see us, with no question, no mention of the bleeding. Could she have forgotten so quickly that I had been bleeding? I mean, look: let's say you see even a complete stranger bleeding on the street, you stop and you hand him a Kleenex (or if you happen to have a spare one on you, a gauze pad) with the expectation that that will help him stop the bleeding, you leave, and five minutes later, bump into him; aren't you going at least to wonder out loud about the bleeding?)

By the way, the following week I mention this bleeding incident to Charlie, who says, "Just to make sure, let's do a clotting test." I go to the lab and the test is done. Forget high tech, forget lasers, forget MRI's! The very good natured, pleasant young woman technician very gently makes a tiny cut in my arm and, stop-watch in one hand, blotting paper in the other, times how long it takes for the bleeding to stop! Anyway, my bleeding, this many days after having stopped aspirin and Plavix, stops in time for the clotting to be considered well within the normal limits, maybe at the fast end.

This, you are probably aware, is only the second time in my saga that I am subjected to a long wait and for that I am very grateful. Once, on a committee for outpatient services at the medical school, I found out that most of the outpatient clinics there gave patients appointments for

9:00 AM or for 1:00 PM and it was first come, first served within those times. The justification was that patients come late and, with every one supposed to be there at the same time, there is some assurance that there are always people in the waiting room to be seen. The argument against that, of course, is that maybe the reason people come late is that they know that if they come on time they will have to wait a long time.

Our committee had the authority to prohibit that kind of scheduling and we legislated instead hourly appointments in all clinics. Most interesting is that, despite an initial outcry, there were no complaints from departments about this new policy after it had been in operation for a while. And yet in the real world habits die slowly. So remember please, that if you are given a medical appointment for 9:00 AM or at 1:00 PM, beware; check out what it means, that is, ask whoever gives you the appointment how many other people have been scheduled for that time, but ask nicely.

Once, the year before she died, Sandra got an appointment to see, for the first time, the Big Hodgkin's Disease Expert at Stanford, the man whose work had been quoted to us now for more than twenty years. We got there on time for our nine o'clock appointment, waited a while in the waiting room, and were then taken to an examining room where we sat by ourselves, nerves completely frayed, until 1:00 PM, when finally our renowned Expert, wearing a white coat, entered the area with a group of students who virtually filled the room.

During the examination and the review of all the material we brought with us and the findings of other Stanford physicians who had seen Sandra some weeks before, the Expert spoke, actually lectured, maybe pontificated is more accurate, almost exclusively to his students—like we just happened to be there. The whole thing was a terribly demeaning experience—waiting for four hours and then being treated like we were animals in a zoo. It was made even more terrible, in retrospect, as it turns out, that the Expert's thinking about the case was quite wrong and led to incorrect treatment! I don't actually blame him for making the error; her medical situation was, at this point in her life, one year before she died, very complex. What I do resent is his performance as God and then being wrong.

Now back to my story. Soon into the room comes the Gastroenterologist, a robust man, somewhat leaner than his face would suggest (I'll bet he recently lost a lot of weight), who looks like he's all heart and, though appreciably younger than I, is the image of everyone's benevolent uncle. He quickly goes through what seems like his repertoire to put us at ease: a few words in Yiddish (always a comfort, right?), questions about where we come from, followed by attempts to communicate familiarity with those cities after perhaps two or three day visits. He doesn't get that *empathic* doesn't mean *seductive*—but I'm cool: at least he's trying. He's wearing dark pants, clearly from a suit, white shirt and tie, and a white coat.

I hope these digressions are not making you crazy, but what is it with these white coats? It seems no longer a commonplace that physicians wear them—lots of doctors I've seen over the last five years don't, so what is the scoop with those who do? Since they, the coats, are not going to be featured in *Gentleman's Quarterly*, nor can they be used as a defense against giving or getting germs—we know nowadays that white coats worn this way offer extremely limited protection, very likely no more than a sweater or a sport jacket would—nor as a way to stay unsoiled and avoid cleaning bill—i.e., most likely, patients are not, without some notice that will surely enable the doctor to get out of the way or put on a white coat in time, going to do something dreadful to one's new Armani jacket—one wonders about their symbolism.

I do have a hint or two from my old days as faculty in the medical school. I began to notice there that some of my psychiatrist colleagues would put on white coats when they were going outside the Department of Psychiatry for meetings or to consult in other departments or for classroom teaching. It seemed to me that what was at issue there was a need on the part of these psychiatrists, in some unmentioned symbolic way, to address the question of their doctorhood, to assert that they were just as much doctors as any of the other specialists; since they never got their hands dirty dealing with patients in any physical way, perhaps they felt a need to prove themselves in this way.

Another hint was when I noticed years ago, giving a talk to a group of psychologists in another medical school, that, in that setting, they (the psychologists), who made a very decent living by charging private fees for services for psychological testing, for example, in neurology and psychiatry departments, were wearing, even at this talk of mine, white coats. It was as though they needed to demonstrate to their medical center colleagues that they were as professional, as "doctoral" as anyone else.

So, very likely the value of white coats when conducting regular office visits is to indicate to the patient that the doctor is of a different status in the relationship, that patient and doctor are not peers, that reciprocity of any kind is not to be expected here. This is a very interesting conjecture to me, because the only two doctors who appear in my saga here who wear white coats routinely are those who do not talk on the phone, who assign the job of communicating afterwards to somebody else. Coincidence? I think not! Well, it's worth thinking about and checking out, isn't it?

We talk, the gastroenterologist and I, about my recent history some, he tsk-tsks appropriately, then asks me to lie on my left side so that he can do a rectal examination to see if there's blood in my stool. The set-up is the traditional one: you lie on a padded table that has a piece of paper pulled over it (to make sure, I guess, that you don't soil the plastic upholstered covering—plastic, in the first place, to prevent any problems; just wash it off and it's as clean as the day it was put on—or use fabric—but without the paper you wouldn't have all the crunching, the bunching up of the paper, and the feeling it gives you that even here you're screwing up, you're making a mess, your skin is even touching the plastic—and when you get off the table, you have to ignore the bunched up ball or insane 3-D ribbon the paper has become, more than likely by now on the floor).

Diana opts to leave the room at this point. With his finger poised to go up my ass, I comment that I hate this now-almost-five-year-long situation, that prior to five years ago I'd always seen myself more as a caregiver than what this situation has allowed. I'm musing, it's meant rhetorically, but he says, as he now withdraws his finger, "Do you want to talk to me more about that now?" Well, of course I don't! I was just making a comment. Why suddenly this psychotherapy mode? And wearing a white coat yet! Is it in medical school or is it in "continuing education" courses that these people learn to come out with lines like this at moments like this? But, enough! This man is trying to do the right thing, to treat me like a person. That's doing more than some.

He tells me to get dressed, leaves the room (you have noticed, I'm sure, that doctors seem unable to tolerate you in the process of dressing or undressing? They don't have problems with you naked or very scantily clad, but the act of removing or putting on clothing seems to be too personal or obscene to be allowed in their presence. It's the action itself that seems off-putting to them. My theory is that in the act of dressing or undressing, your personhood, your humanity cannot be denied—you are someone doing something—I move, therefore I am. Naked you can be an object) and comes back with the news that indeed there is blood and we ought to look to find out where it's coming from by scheduling a colonoscopy and endoscopy. "We'll find it for you," he says reassuringly, like Superman vowing to rid Gotham City of evil. You've got to hand it to the guy, he's always trying; he rarely gets it right, but he does try. He tells me to go to Maria, that she will set up the appointment for me.

I go to Maria as I have been told to do, but first, of course, I have to find out which of the four women in the office she is! I try one and it is she. In addition to the appointment, she is to give me a prescription for the laxative I'm to take in preparation for the endoscopy and colonoscopy (*prepare* is the euphemism for the h-bomb type action of the laxative; a half gallon mixture—they give you a little packet of flavoring to add, but, trust me, nothing helps; the problem is not entirely the taste, the texture figures in also—to be drunk the night before the procedure, eight ounces at a time, every thirty minutes: if you close your eyes, think about something else, and swallow fast, it's just barely tolerable) and also a sheet of paper with directions (directions for the laxative and to the Endoscopy Center are on the same sheet of paper; a direction, after all, is a direction). The instructions indicate that the procedures are done in Room 103 in the hospital, but the little map shows only where the building is, not where the rooms are in the building, and I do know that the numbering system within the main hospital building can sometimes be tricky. I ask Maria where Room 103 might be and she says that it is right near the Emergency Room.

Of course, right in line with our newly learned expectations, Maria doesn't give me the appointment for my two-act production right then; it's just not done that way. Later, when I'm not around, she will call the Endoscopy center to make the appointment (apparently it is against the rules for this kind of transaction, a phone call between two gate keepers, to be done in front of a patient; perhaps the patient might learn something that he/she ought not to know) and then, the following day, I am supposed to call her and she will give me the time and day that I'm scheduled for, one week later.

You might notice in the way that this interaction is set up that my schedule is of absolutely no interest, it has no relevance to the task at hand; I might have plans to lunch with the President, maybe I'm supposed to be at The Meeting that will finally stop war and end world poverty forever, maybe Ava Gardner is back and we are to have dinner, but nobody asks. Reciprocity is not a value here. I am to show up when and where they tell me to, having, as they say, "prepared" myself the day before and without anything to eat since lunchtime the day of the "preparation"—although it would surely have been difficult anyway to eat anything with that "preparation" taking place.

I get to the hospital in time enough for my appointment, enter through the main door, and head off toward the emergency room—that's what Maria told me, right? I notice that I'm passing numbers close to 120 and that they're getting higher. And then I notice a sign on the wall saying *Endoscopy* with an arrow that points in the direction opposite to my route. Never to be considered rigid, I turn around, retrace my steps, and go off in the opposite direction, away from the Emergency Room, and eventually down a strangely lit, somewhat littered corridor, and, off to one side; we find it (maybe Maria is right after all—maybe this is the back end of the ER, where the ambulances drive up, but how would someone in my position know that).

It's called *The Endoscopy Center*, that is what the signs say; I guess that they are a bit embarrassed that they do colonoscopies too? There is less gentility apparently in shoving tubes up your ass than in shoving them down your throat. And here I've been noticing for a while that colonoscopies are all the rage these days; they've certainly been getting a lot of press.

Once there, everyone who deals with me in the Endoscopy Center is particularly nice, kind, empathic, even smart, even adult, ready with all the information I ask for, and never condescending. I'm taken to what seems like an examining room, a very engaging nurse tells me what's going to happen in one of the least patronizing manners that my saga has thus far afforded, sets up an IV and she says that soon it's going to seem to me that I'm asleep, though I'll be able to react to what they ask me.

My gastroenterologist comes in, he is very pleasant and, thankfully, business-like, there is no occasion for Yiddish this time in our very brief interaction, this time it's only business, there is very little patter of any kind, there is no need to do those reassuring bits now, it all seems very fast, and the next thing I know, I'm in something like a recovery room. And after all that prodding, there is no pain, no discomfort, at the most maybe a little bloating for a couple of days, but nothing at all to cringe or complain about!

Let me tell you what they did to me while I was unconscious. First, the nurse assured me that it will feel to me like unconsciousness and I will remember nothing, but that actually I will follow orders during the procedure, like I will swallow when they tell me to. You all know probably that an endoscopy amounts to a tube going down your esophagus and into your stomach, transmitting images of what's what there. A colonoscopy is its complement: a tube going, via the rectum, all the way to the end (no, really to the beginning) of the large bowel. These tubes are very nifty contraptions: they not only transmit images, they wash the linings, if needed, they clip little pieces for biopsies, if needed—they are your all purpose tubes!

It's Monday. As we leave, they tell Diana and me to call on Friday, that very likely the report will be in by then. So we call on Friday and are told that the nurse practitioner (*NP*, from now on) is not there right now. Interesting, isn't it, that the message clearly is that we speak to the *NP*, not to the doctor, the man who talks with us in Yiddish and waxes nostalgic about where we grew up (like we're from the same shtetl). The rules here, though more structured, are like those in Vascular Surgery. Roles here, though not described out loud, are clearly delineated—the role of the physician is again not to talk with his patients, at least not on the phone. Is it that his time can be used better otherwise? Or does he do this (i.e., talk on the phone) badly? Or is talking to patients a lower order of things that physicians ought not to be doing?

Whatever the reasons for this distribution of labor, we ask that someone—anyone—please call us later in the day, even if only to tell us that the report has not yet come in. She agrees and promises that that will be done. I am sure that I do not surprise those of you who have followed my adventures of the previous five years when I tell you that nobody calls. We call the office at 4:00PM and the answering service tells us that the office closed at 3:30.

The weekend, as you might imagine, is rather long. But we manage to smile through. We call on Monday and again are told that the *NP* is not in and, after much coaxing, that the report too is not yet in. I offer to call the pathologist and check things out myself, but she says that no, they will certainly take care of it, in a timely fashion. I point out that this is a problem for me, what ought I to do now, a full week after the procedure, to find out whether or not I have a malignancy? (because, though it's never been mentioned, that is what we are all worried about, right?)—"Certainly," I say, "people in your office would not be comfortable in a situation like you all have placed me in."

I feel heartless putting her into this defensive position—the situation I find myself in is certainly not her doing and I don't want to kill or hurt the messenger—but I have to express how desperate I am beginning to feel, in the hope that this desperation of mine will light a fire that will enable her to convince someone to speak with me and tell me something; I'll even settle for "Sorry." "Hope springs eternal", as they say, and I'm afraid I don't learn well from experience

She says that she will page the *NP* who will call me; she adds that the *NP* will not be in the next day and that the day after that the office is closed for a national holiday. "That means," I tell her, "that the results of my tests will not be available to me for 10 days after the procedure." She acknowledges that that would be unfortunate and says again that she will page the *NP*, who will certainly be calling us.

Five hours later, since we've not heard from the *NP*, Diana calls them. The secretary is surprised at our news and tells Diana that she will page the *NP* right then and that we can speak with her directly. After literally ten minutes on hold, Maria gets back on the line (imagine the conversation between her and the *NP*!) to say that the biopsies are not in yet (see, apparently there is a rule that we were not aware of: *NP*s do not talk with you unless biopsies are in), so there's no reason really to speak with the *NP*, but otherwise the colonoscopy is normal (what about the endoscopy?)—except for a hiatal hernia in the esophagus (isn't that information from the endoscopy?), which we've known about since my first CT scan five years ago, there is a node in a place that I never even heard of (and I don't know how to find out about without hours of phone tag and feeling put down), and a polyp in the colon (not too bad a thing, I feel: it puts me up there with recent American presidents). I do not know what all this means: for example, what did they biopsy? what is it we are waiting for? But it's absolutely clear now that I am driving office personnel here crazy and that I won't know anything until Thursday. The *NP* has obviously struck her pose and will not budge.

Right? Wrong! In fact, she, the *NP* herself, calls on Wednesday (could it be that I'd made Maria so nervous that she reversed days in communicating to us the business of days off? After all, Tuesday, it turns out, was a holiday, so likely the office was closed, and on Wednesday, perhaps the *NP* had changed her plans and decided to come in. Whatever the reasons, I'm taken aback and have to give up a little of my paranoia. Life keeps me on my toes), nine days after the procedure, to say that the pathology report has just come in and that everything looks "good," the biopsies show that everything is benign, but that, because of the node and the polyp, I ought to have another endoscopy and colonoscopy in three years. (In three years? As my mother used to say, "I should only live so long!") Amen! "So, then," I ask, "why the bleeding and anemia?" "Oh!" she says. "Right! Oh, well, let me speak to the doctor and we can set up another test to check out your small intestine."

Not bloody likely! Am I hearing right? Wasn't it their job to find the source of bleeding somewhere in my gastro-intestinal system? Isn't that the reason that we undertook this procedure? Didn't the doctor say to me, "We'll find it for you?" Instead of "Why the hell didn't you look there when you had me 'prepared' and on the table?" I mumble something non-committal, and then days later, when Maria calls (notice that it's not the *NP*—the *NP* calls apparently only about results, not appointments) to set something up, I say, "Well, not now, maybe later," because I refuse to care about my small intestine, I've got better things to do! My hemoglobin is up (for the first time in five years it's within the normal range), on a recent rectal exam there is no evidence of blood, and I feel healthy.

I learn some weeks later that, as a result of my putting off any further tests, the gastroenterology office calls Charlie—he is, after all, the referrer—to let him know what I did and, best of all, to find out if my putting things off is OK with him, like they're squealing on me and he's going to make me do something I do not want to do: fat chance! Whatever they say, I certainly will not follow up, at least not for a while, not until I myself decide that I ought to and when it will be done. I cannot let anyone push me around medically. I need to feel like an autonomous human being. Life is too good to give up that sweet, precious autonomy; and, in fact, for me, it is that precious autonomy that allows life to be so good. It makes me sing all day long. I am Gene Kelly, singing in the rain, and I would be a fool to give that up.

Later

So, four and a half years after they told me that in three years I was to have another endoscopy and colonoscopy, I call to make an appointment, and, after some considerable time apparently looking up records, the person I am speaking with chides me that I was supposed to return in a year for an endoscopy. I say that nobody had ever told me that; and, fearing some retribution because I am a year and a half late (never mind the attempt that I had made two and a half years after the first time, an attempt denied me because it was less than three years), I add that the time frame I was given was three years. Silence on the phone: could she be worrying about legal issues if indeed what I am reporting is true? And then a recovery, i.e. she gives me an appointment for two months later. Could this two month delay be punishment for my year and a half procrastination? She takes some information, all of which is available on the computer, says she will send me some material, and the call ends.

A few days later, I realize that I have a prior appointment elsewhere on the scheduled day, call back, and speak with a different woman, who quickly rearranges a new appointment. The following week, I get two packets in the mail, one, it turns out, from each of the women I spoke with, with appointment information (this is what shows me that each is from one of the women on the phone), a prescription for the "preparation," and, in each, a form to be filled out listing the drugs I take. Four weeks later I receive an identical packet, though this time there is the statement that there is a new time for the appointment, the time I arranged with the second woman I spoke with. Well, it's always nice to get mail.

The day before the appointment, at four in the afternoon, I begin the preparation; every ten minutes, I am to drink eight ounces of the clear liquid I've made by adding warm water to the powder in the gallon plastic jug I have paid (they tell me that my insurance won't cover it) $37.50 for at the drugstore (the liquid, the consistency of Jello before it gels, and smelling faintly of pineapple, one of the five flavorings I can choose to add). Eight ounces of anything every ten minutes seems a lot to swallow, but imagine dealing with something of this consistency and faint aroma. I do manage to get it all but about an inch of it down before the vomiting starts. Now the whole house smells faintly of pineapple, but the clean-up could have been a lot worse. At this point in my "preparation,'" there is nothing left in me to vomit, so it's all "the preparation" itself. Needless to say, however, the liquid does its job: sick to my stomach, I am clear as a bell.

The appointment time is eleven, but in each of my three packets, it says that I should arrive an hour before the appointment. I know that it will take perhaps five minutes to take care of whatever business they want me to set aside an hour for, but no matter how slowly I try to drive to the hospital, I am in the reception area exactly at ten. The waiting area is a truncated right triangle, the entrance and reception desk at the truncation and its narrow end. There is just enough room between the desk and the wall for one person to stand facing the desk. Moving to or from the area is a rather awkward maneuver, because there is not enough room to be perpendicular to the desk and wall. But we manage.

There is one person ahead of me; within five minutes, his business is concluded, I have handed in my list of drugs, answered the two or three questions I am asked (all of the answers, by the way, are in my file or in the computer), I have listened to the receptionist's spiel (sotto voce) about the dreadful things that can happen, signed consent forms, and I am sitting, staring into space, at five after ten. What does the fact that I am required to come an hour prior to my appointment and wait fifty five minutes of that hour supposed to mean about me in relation to the doctor and the institution? Well first, my time has no value. The status of patient somehow obviates this value for me. That I am to sit there with nothing to do, for no reason, must surely indicate a reduction of my personhood in the eyes of those who run this shop. They could have asked me to come in ten minutes before the hour if I or my time had any significance, but, trust me, as you will see, it gets worse.

Since the only magazines in the basket are Women's Day (the person sitting beside me grabbed Vanity Fair just as I was going to reach for it), I continue in my space staring posture until about five to eleven, when I am called out of the reception area and taken to a changing room: a room with many lockers, small dressing rooms, piles of hospital garments ("put this one on, open in the back, and this one over it, open in the front, and these socks"), a couple of bathrooms (a lucky thing because I have become obsessed with the possibility that I have not adequately completed my "preparation," and will cause problems during the colonoscopy). There are actually lockers along two short walls; along one, the lockers have no keys (signifying, I think, that people are using these lockers and have the keys with them) along the other, about half have keys. During my short wait, after changing my clothes, I notice that hospital staff comes in to use the toilets, one uses one of the lockers on the wall of lockers without keys and a dressing room and I realize that I am in a democratized area. The changing room is not only co-ed, but used by staff and patients with no discrimination. I am getting subtle, but mixed messages now about the esteem patients obtain here, but there is also some evidence that in the minds of those that designed this set-up, nurses and patients have equal status.

I change my clothing as directed, struggle to lock the locker (I succeed exactly one second before my guide reaches over to show me how), and follow my guide into the recovery room, which serves also as a staging area.

It always gives me great pleasure in hospitals to see those curtains suspended by chains or bead from the ceiling, around beds, because many years ago, after our bathroom was redone, I got the idea visiting Sandra in the hospital after she had broken her elbow in a fall, circle dancing at a bar-mitzva dinner, to suspend the shower curtain from the ceiling, thus getting rid of the need for those tubes that, hanging from the ceiling, with a tube holding the set-up in place at three spots, describe the outline of the tub. It was a major achievement for me to put it up and its invention and execution were for me great sources of pride. And that was the set-up here, not around tubs, of course, but around gurneys. I am ushered into one of the cubicles defined by curtains, get up on a gurney, have my vital signs taken (my blood pressure, as a result of Avastin and my reaction to the indignity of coming an hour early is higher than it's ever been) am set up with an IV for hydration and there I lie. Every so often a new nurse comes in and introduces herself as my nurse; I guess that the short tenure of my nurses has to do with the lunch schedule and my long wait.

After an hour or so, my gurney is pushed into a small room across the hallway, the nurse of the moment chats with me with some ease and interest, and when she leaves, I realize that because they have pushed me in feet first, the back of my head is at the door, and though I hear voices in the hallway I can see only the top of the doorway reflected in the glass door of a cabinet opposite the door, high enough so that nothing in the hallway is reflected. I am about to get claustrophobic from the stimulus deprivation about twenty minutes into this, when a young man arrives, introduces himself as a "fellow" (I never suspected him of being a girl), says he's sorry that our main man is late but he is upstairs (in a ten story building, what can upstairs communicate?), and he looks as though he is about to interview me. I ask whether he thinks that his apology and the man's being upstairs (as far as I am concerned he could be upstairs sleeping!) are supposed to obviate the rudeness of his now being an hour and twenty minutes late. He says, "No," begins to interview me, and it becomes clear that this young man still retains humor and empathy. When I tell him that I had been on the faculty of the University of Illinois Medical School for many years, he responds that he knows the institution, having gotten a Bachelor's and a medical degree at Northwestern. I comment on my long and complex relationship with Northwestern and we are now like old buddies, about to have a beer. He laughs at my jokes, the interview style is dropped, he finds ways to touch my shoulder, my upper arm; the room is aquiver with warmth and affection, and then he has to leave.

Now it is twelve thirty five, an hour and thirty five minutes after the appointment, two hours and thirty five minutes of waiting. Soon a nurse comes in, we chat about her work, I complain about the wait, she is most reasonable, open, and intelligent in her responses, and time passes. At one, she indicates that the doctor has come in and that she will get me ready by giving me medication. Her tone indicates that the medication is going to put me to sleep and if I remember from four and a half years back it acts fast; I ask her to put it off a few minutes, so I can speak with the doctor before the procedure. "Oh," she says, "you want to speak with him before the procedure," as if it's quite a novelty to want to speak with someone one hasn't seen for four and a half years and who is about to invade my ass. I am not intimidated, she makes a phone call, and goes about her business.

After a few moments, I hear a voice behind me saying, "Hello, my friend ('my friend' yet—I wouldn't make a friend of mine wait two hours for me). How are you doing?" (No comment about his lateness, no apology, no nothing, as though it's customary for patients to accept this degree of lateness.) I respond, "Not too well." He comes into my vision to ask what the problem is, and although I have promised myself that I will say nothing critical prior to the procedure, I blurt out, "Well, I've been waiting for you for two hours." He says, and this is the full quote, "Oh, I'm sorry." No excuse, no "I was debauching upstairs" or "I overslept" or "The dog ate my homework" Nothing. Nada.

I then bring up what my oncologist asked that I speak with him about: to keep in mind that I am on Avastin (more about that later), which likely has an effect on my healing, because there will likely be a need for biopsies. He says that he will be as careful as he can be, things will be all right, and the next thing I know, I'm waking up in the recovery room. I ask a nurse if I'm going to see the doctor, and she says,

"No. He's gone," which means, I guess, that had I not asked to see him prior to the procedure, I would not see him at all; had I not met him four and a half years ago, I would not even know what he looks like! I also learn that it's three o'clock, that I've been in the recovery area fifty minutes, sleeping, that nothing untoward showed up in either procedure (except for a hiatal hernia which I learned about from a CT scan nine and a half years ago and a hemorrhoid that I and my oncologist predicted several weeks ago).

I don't quite get this: four and a half years ago I had both a polyp and a node and now nothing. I thought that those sorts of things are supposed to get worse, so where did they go? And he too is gone, and from my experience last time I know that I will not be able to speak with him directly on the phone. So, can I ever know what's really going on? Since I now know that the tests have essentially negative results, there is apparently no need for biopsies (or is the decision not to biopsy a result of caution in relation to the Avastin—we'll never know, will we), and thus I have all the information that I will have and won't need to call him for more, so, without having said good-by, my relationship with this almost invisible doctor is over.

I look up and see that Diana has entered the area, I sing a few bars of *A Pretty Girl is Like a Melody*, she tells me to quiet down, is ushered out and told to wait for me in the changing room; I get out of bed (you can't say, "out of gurney"), one of the nurses helps me out of the room, I get my clothes from my locker, change where I had changed before, we (Diana and I) walk to the building's entrance, and Diana leaves me to get the car. After a few minutes, in relation to what is known in Yiddish as shpilkes (in English: I can't sit still), I leave the lobby, wait outside, Diana drives up, and home we go.

The following morning I notice that the area just under my chest hurts like hell. It is as though I am bruised inside and that is certainly understandable with the endoscopy tube having been shoved down my throat, down my esophagus, into my stomach, and then my duodenum. My fantasy, of course, is that the gastroenterologist, enraged that I called him on his lateness, got even by taking extra care to bruise the hell out of me. I dismiss this rationally, remembering that on two previous occasions, when tubes were placed down there, there was pain for a few days—and yet I am able to relish the fantasies. Of course, I tell no one. The pain lasts three or four days. Nobody has warned me of discomfort following the procedure.

The procedures were done on a Monday and it was suggested that I call on Friday to get the results, but as I said there is no point in calling since the nurse indicated that there are no untoward findings. And yet I cannot resist the call; I need to hear how they are going to present whatever they want to tell me. So, on Monday, two weeks after the procedure, I call. The excuse I give is that I want to make sure that a report will be sent to Dr. Caplin, my primary physician; their records indicate that that has already been taken care of and would I like the nurse practitioner (*NP*) to call me to discuss the results with me? I figure, "Why not?.' and say that I would like that and would also like the results faxed to me; she agrees that they can fax them, but only after I've spoken with the *NP*. She also says that the *NP* will call me in one or two days.

Two days later (not one day; two days), the *NP* calls. She tells me that a hiatal hernia was found (a first clue that the report from four and a half years ago is ignored), no polyps, no nodes no comment about where they had gone in the last four and a half years (a second clue to the ignoring of the earlier report). She starts to mention some findings, but, apparently puzzled by them, stops and wonders about the state of my liver. While I am picking myself up off the floor, I remember that blood results of liver functions, the CT scans, and MRI's too all indicate that my liver is essentially problem-free; I tell her that, she changes the subject. She tells me that "he" (the gastroenterologist is never referred to by name, title, or profession during this conversation, he is always *he*:perhaps we might capitalize the *H*) wants to repeat the endoscopy in a year, I ask why, she says, after a long delay (perusing, no doubt, my previous write-up), because of the polyp and node, I say they are gone now, and she goes on to the next subject. I ask her to fax me the report, she says she will, and it arrives within a half hour.

IX

*In which I learn that there may or there may not be
a number of ways to skin a cat, if you are able to
find the cat*

So, everything's good: no pain, no shortness of breath.
I can walk wherever I want, and soon, even my PCR is
completely negative for the Philadelphia chromosome
(that is, there is no way to detect any remnant of leukemia
in my body). Life, as they say, is sweet

Two and a half years after my colonoscopy, at an annual
visit to Richard Caplin, we decide that it would be a good
idea to have a CT scan; it's now seven and a half years since
the nephrectomy, so it's doubtful that any metastases will
show up, but better safe than sorry. So an appointment is
arranged and I go in. This time I don't have to drink anything,
I don't have to dress any particular way, I am just to be
there ten minutes before the procedure in order to fill out
some forms. Everything goes according to plan, they lead
me into the scan room, I get up on the table, they make a
big deal about the fact that because I have only one kidney
they cannot inject the contrast (which is metabolized in the
kidney and can therefore do my remaining one damage),
they haphazardly cover me with a blanket while asking that
I lower my pants a bit, and we're off.

When it's over, I'm sitting on the table, and I surprise even myself when I say, "When the radiologist reads this, I'd like to talk to him." The technicians look aghast, as though my request is the most outlandish thing they've ever heard and one of them says, "Well, he's very busy." I reply that I am aware of that, but that I would like, nonetheless, to speak with him if I may. They lead me back to the waiting room, saying that they will see what they can do. I'm sitting there maybe five minutes when one of the technicians comes to me and says, like he's meeting Gandhi, that the radiologist would like to talk with me. He leads me to a phone, I pick up and the radiologist asks if I've been having any pain. (Well here goes. The day had started so nice and now I'm in for it!) I say, "No," and then very cleverly, "Why do you ask?" He explains that since they were not able to use contrast, things are not very clear, but there is something suspicious; it looks like there is a mass on my pancreas. (Pancreas! I don't even know where it is. What I do know is that my father and Sydney Berg, whose bar mitzvah ceremony took place with mine, both died of pancreatic cancer. We have discovered a cancer that's very likely going to kill me, but at least I got the guy to talk to me.

He says he will contact Richard Caplin, the referrer, to decide how to get a better fix on what these cloudy "masses" are: MRI, sonogram, God knows what, and I go home. I call Richard's office immediately and he very quickly calls me back. He says that the radiologist did not think it was pancreatic cancer, if anything it is more probably metastases of the kidney cancer removed in the nephrectomy seven and a half years ago (this degree of specificity from a cloudy image that needs confirmation through a new procedure!). He says that his office will mail me a referral for an MRI and the phone number of the office that makes appointments and that, as a courtesy, he will send a copy of the radiologist's report to my kidney surgeon,

The referral comes in the mail the next day and I call to set up the appointment. The next appointment available is two and a half weeks hence; despite my view that the cancer will probably have killed me by then, I make the appointment. Two or three days later, I get a phone call from a woman who identifies herself by her first name, as being from the kidney surgeon's office; she says the he would like me to see a different surgeon (a pancreas man, I take it) in the office and that that person's secretary (also identified by her first name) will be in touch with me in a couple of days. When I tell her that I don't know what this is for, she gets nervous, reiterates that so and so will be calling me, and that's that. And, indeed, the next day, so and so calls. By this time I have figured out that the kidney surgeon has interpreted the courtesy radiology report as a referral to him and he is taking charge. He is my nemesis, and he is taking charge. I explain that because of one kidney, and therefore no contrast, the CT scan is unclear and I have arranged for an MRI two weeks hence. She puts me on hold and Susan takes over. In a very loud, strident voice, a voice that forces me to move the phone away from my ear, she tells me that two weeks is a long time, asks if the referral has been made by some one on the university faculty, and when I say, "No," says that she is sure that she can get an earlier appointment. I ask that she not do that (I do not want privileges of rank), she acquiesces and sets up an appointment for me to see the new surgeon on a Thursday, two days after the MRI, so the surgeon will have had a chance to check out the films.

My appointment for the MRI is on a Tuesday at 3:30. I get a call on Monday asking that I be there a half hour early to do forms and whatever. I get there then at 3:00 and there is no one at the desk. I sign in and a few minutes later, there are three women, clearly employees, circulating around the desk, dealing with people, shuffling papers, ignoring me. After about 20 minutes, my name is called, I go to the desk, and am asked to fill out a form, essentially a list of man-made items that may be in my body that will interfere with the magnetic functions of the MRI. Since I have none, I finish the check-list in less than 2 minutes, bring it up to the desk and sit. At 3:40, I approach the desk and am told that the technicians are still with the previous patient. At 3:55, I am called out and told that they are ready for me now; I am taken to a locker area, asked to change into a hospital Johnny coat (but to keep my shoes and socks on—quite a look). When I've changed, I'm to wait (for10 minutes) on a bench. At 4:05, I am approached by a technician, and we are on our way.

There are horror movies that begin to convey the feeling of being in the MRI set-up, once you're moved into the machine, but for my money, Vincent Price doesn't come close. My technician has placed earphones on me, I think to distract me from the physical situation with "easy" rock music and to enable me to hear her commands about taking deep breaths and letting them go. The banality of the music, however, distracts me from nothing. My technician has told me that the procedure lasts about forty five minutes, but once I'm slid into the tube (so tight that I can barely raise my head or move my arms outward), I'm afraid I cannot last that long in there. She has given me a rubber bulb to press if there is an emergency (that is, if the closeness becomes unbearable) and I know that she can hear me if I say anything. Those two things plus shut eyes and the ability to project parts of movies in my head get me through. When I open my eyes and see a vertical row of lights just inches from my face, my need to keep my eyes closed is strongly reinforced. I am also able to forestall panic by rehearsing how I might ask her to change the radio station to one that features jazz or classical music; I never do it, but the exercise is useful and I survive

When I'm slid out of the apparatus, I comment that I do get claustrophobic in rooms, crowded with people moving around, but surprisingly I managed in this horror. She says, "I guess you can ride in planes. I can't." Rather than discuss the irony (or sadism) of her subjecting other people to what panics her, I allow the subject to drop, change my clothes, and leave. You will notice that this time I do not ask to speak to the radiologist; with probabilities of positive results having been raised by the cloudy images on the CT scan, I don't want to take my chance of hearing bad news just to prove a point. But when I get home I call Caplin and he says that the MRI confirms the impression of the CT scan that there is a mass on my pancreas and that everyone involved thinks it's a metastasis from the kidney cancer, rather than a new primary pancreatic cancer.

Two days later we arrive for our 1:00 PM appointment with the surgeon. It's the same waiting-area where we waited several years ago for the vascular surgeon, with those huge columns that preclude one's keeping an eye on the people at the desk or them on you. It's not a Monday, so no vascular people are there. I very quickly fill out the forms they want me to fill out, and after a short while, we are escorted to an examining room, where there are three chairs and an examining table. Which two of the three seats are we to sit on? Although Diana aims for the chair with arms at the writing table, I caution her that that is very likely reserved for the doctor, and we both sit on armless chairs. Soon, the woman who led us to the room enters and says that the doctor is here, but is reading my file now. I do not raise the question of why my appointment was not arranged for when he will have finished reviewing the material. (You may think that she came in with this news as a response to my making my impatience noticed. No, no, no. This time it is lovely Diana who has begun to pace the halls),

Soon into the room come a young Asian man, white jacketed, meticulously groomed, extremely clean, very good-looking and a younger woman who remains in the background. He introduces himself as Dr. Kim and her as a student (if she's a student, what the hell is he?); he takes a seat and begins the interview. Initially a bit stiff, he quickly relaxes, listens to and laughs at my stories. He asks the usual questions (eg. What am I allergic to?) and I give my answers, direct, but layered, ironic, and textured with whatever craziness the story affords. I can't help it, but he seems to like the act. When his questions have been dealt with, he asks to see the scar from my nephrectomy and I am pleased to unbutton my shirt and comment on its size. Ready to leave, he says that he and the student will talk to the surgeon, tell him what they've learned and then he, the surgeon, will be in to see me.

So we wait, Diana pacing the halls and I a bit more restrained. After about twenty minutes, we hear them coming. First the surgeon, introducing himself, hand extended to shake mine, followed by Kim and the student. The surgeon looks rather like editors of newspapers used to look in black and white movies (Technicolor movies, you may have noticed, do not often have editors and when they do, it's Jason Robards) and he's almost scowling, but he's not wearing a white coat and he has on a tie with small figures randomly but closely printed on a blue field, very much like a flowered tie I have, so I'm prepared to like him.

He says that indeed the MRI shows what Richard had told me, but he adds that there are three nodules and with his thumb and forefinger he shows that the size is of a large grape. He says that very likely he will need to take out the pancreas and that I will then be diabetic and have digestive problems, all controllable with drugs. I ask if the nodes can be excised, with most of the pancreas remaining and he agrees and expresses some pleasure that we can avoid the diabetes and digestive problems. (So why the hell did he come up with removing the entire pancreas to begin with? Taking out seems to be a disease these people have!) We chat a bit about possibilities, I mention the idea of aliens, like with John Hurt in *Alien*, we talk about what might happen if left alone, and he reassures me that, unlike Sydney Berg and my father, I will not die of pancreatic cancer, because that is not what this is. He cracks a smile now and then, but quickly returns to the near scowl.

The plan he has worked out is that I will see a medical oncologist (he tells me his name) and that we will then confer about what we do next; now there will be a team and God knows everyone likes a team. We are told to wait in the waiting room for *Susan* to set up the appointment with the oncologist or at least get us the phone number.

After about 20 minutes (Diana still pacing, even asking at the desk for Susan), out comes Susan (it's the same voice I heard on the phone) who says that the surgeon had spoken with the kidney surgeon and that plans have changed some (I am sure you notice who is left out of the planning): I am to have blood work done immediately, go to the radiation library where I will pick up a CD of all my material, she will fax what she has to the person at another hospital who does *INTERVENTIONAL ENDOSCOPY* (she says it as though it is all capitalized—it is a procedure whereby a biopsy and sonogram of the nodules can be made with a needle and whatever is used for sonograms attached to the same sort of contraption used in a regular endoscopy), and that person's office will call me to make an appointment for the procedure; when the results of the procedure are ready I will have a meeting with the kidney surgeon to decide if the next step is surgery of medical oncology. I am fine with all that, it seems a better plan; I just wonder how the changes got made and what that means organizationally, etc. But I'm easy.

I go down to the lab, take a number, Diana goes to deal with the car which we were lucky enough to park on the street, to make sure we don't get a parking ticket, I race over to the radiation library across the street, lab number in my hand, and even though I'd been given the wrong room number for the library, find it quickly, sign for the CD, and meet Diana back at the lab, my number not yet having been called. Very soon, blood is drawn and we go home.

By 4:00 the next day, Friday, I've not heard from the interventional endoscopy people, so I call Susan, who had told me to call should there be any problems. I explain the situation when she calls back in response to my message and she tells me (although it sounds like she's shouting at me) that she just faxed them the material and that it will take them about two business days to get back to me (*two business days*: like I'm dealing with some—what shall I call it—business, like the phone company).

So Tuesday, late in the afternoon (two business days, right?), Diana takes matters into her own hands and calls the interventional endoscopy people. After some misdialing and rather strange communications, she gets the person responsible for scheduling and that person looks me up and says that they just received the faxed material (remember, Susan told me Friday afternoon that she had just faxed the material and here it is late Tuesday afternoon and they just got it—oh, the marvels of the information age) and it will be a day or two before the doctor can review it and they will call me then. Thursday afternoon, I get the call; she tells me that an appointment has been set up for the following Thursday (now two weeks after initiating an attempt to make the appointment), at 8:30AM and that I'm to come in an hour early (here we go again: arrive an hour early to wait). This time, I'm sure that you have noticed that the appointment is made with no concern about my schedule, my sleeping habits; my life style.

We get the endoscopy done. Despite the comments of the nurse beforehand, that I will be conscious during the procedure, I remember nothing, but I'm reminded of it the next day, because I feel like I've been kicked in the chest and belly and acid reflux has returned with a vengeance. It's small potatoes, but no one warned me and my unconsciousness precludes any stories.

I am supposed to call the kidney surgeon to set up a meeting. Diana calls and leaves a message when we get home Thursday. Since they don't return the call, I call again Friday mid-afternoon and leave a message. A couple of hours later, I get a call from the very warm, supportive, empathic doctor who did the endoscopy, to say that the cytology results were in and that the tumor is indeed a metastasis of the seven and a half year ago renal cell carcinoma. I suppose that it's a bad thing to have a metastasis of anything, but since everybody I've heard of with pancreatic cancer is dead in a year, I don't know the mortality from metastases of renal cell carcinoma, and so long as I don't know, I'm happy with what I've got and I know that at least for the moment there are no observable (by CT scan and MRI) lesions elsewhere and it's taken seven and a half years to get to this point. We take our joys where we can.

But when is the surgeon going to call me back? And what will my metastatic situation be then? Picture this: I'm in a hurry to get in touch with this schmuck who, in my view, recklessly removed my kidney, lied to me, disfigured me, got rid of me, because he wants a meeting. How much of the planning can I trust him with? My nemesis has my life in his hands.

Alas, the best (and worst) laid plans of mice and men need not always work out. The assistant finally calls me back Monday afternoon; she, very chipper, introduces herself and asks how she can help me. I tell her that I was supposed to set up a meeting with her boss (I'm reading from the note that the pancreas surgeon's assistant gave me), tell her a little of the story, and as soon as I say "pancreas," she says, "Oh, he doesn't do pancreases" (nor windows, I expect). I explain that I am merely doing what he told me to do, she puts me on hold (it's Vivaldi and the cheeriness of the goddamn Four Seasons makes me sick), gets back on in a few minutes and says that the surgeon's nurse practitioner (NP—remember) had just gotten an email from the surgeon and the plan in that email is different from what I've described, but there will continue to be emails exchanged and she will call me about what I am to do. I make it clear to her that I need to hear from her this day.

She calls within the hour and says that *Jerry*, who sets up appointments for the oncology people, will call me to set something up for me to see a medical oncologist. In 20 minutes, Jerry calls, says he's not quite sure which of two urological oncologists I should be seeing (the specialties get finer and finer), but he will take a chance and he gives me an appointment to see one of them in a week; before the transaction is finished, he says that he just received an email from the surgeon (this surgeon is an email freak!)—and he's glad it came, because you've got to listen to a department head—and he, Jerry, was right in the doctor he chose for me. (No "Question authority" here. No doubt Jerry was born after *MASH*, *The Graduate*, and *The Battle of Algiers*)

To me, this is an incredible story. My doctor, out of courtesy, sends the surgeon a report relating to a cancer that he (the surgeon) ostensibly removed (along with a kidney) seven and a half years ago (and told my wife that he'd removed the kidney to prevent the recurrence of the cancer). Immediately the surgeon assumes the role of manager of the case, without ever dealing with me personally, by phone, in his office, whatever. He is managing essentially some spots on an MRI and some cells from a biopsy. And I don't have a say in any of the choices being made! He is unseen and omnipotent. Sounds like some people's idea of God, doesn't it? Could he be? Well, at least those confronting conversations I rehearse at night (instead of sleeping) about the reasons I don't trust him will not take place. Now I can stop rehearsing and perhaps sleep instead.

So, OK. The urological oncologist to whom I'm assigned is Jonathan Rosenberg (the name itself suggests a perfect oncologist for any Jewish mother of an eligible daughter). I look him up on the internet and he has shining qualities galore: young (those are the ones who are up-to-date on everything), Harvard Medical (one block from the high school I went to), reddish hair (one takes pleasure where one can), and prior involvement with Charlie Linker. My prospects now are excellent.

We go in for the appointment. His office is in the Cancer Care Center and even though it has moved a block, it is still the Cancer Center, the one I entered many pages ago, when my saga first began. My reaction this time, however, is different from then; I suppose that that is because I have become a pro at cancer and it's like water off a duck's back. Jonathan is even better than we expected: candid, using big words that he expects us to understand, writes down notes about possible drugs (notes that he wants me to keep), never talks down, not only laughs at my jokes but does a few of his own, a young man, clearly loving his work, up on everything, eager to share, and never talking down. He takes my comments, my questions, my ideas seriously. We are in love.

He talks about the three medications available for my kind of cancer. Two of them are so close to Gleevec in structure and aim that he is reluctant to use them while I am still on Gleevec, and nobody feels that I should be getting off Gleevec. He feels then that the more conservative approach would be a drug called Avastin, manufactured by Genentech and aimed at reducing blood supply to cancer cells and thereby shrinking the cancer. Sounds right to me, at least for the time being, unless we find that Avastin has not done what we hope.

The plan is first to make sure that this tumor is related to the renal cell carcinoma and not the prostate cancer. My job is to get hold of all the biopsy material from a few weeks ago (the procedure was not done at this hospital) and that from the prostate biopsy five years ago; this latter material is in Oklahoma (yes, Oklahoma) and, because it's so old, is in an off-campus storage facility, so it will take up to two weeks to get it. I urge speed because my next appointment with Jonathan is two weeks hence and he plans to have had the pathology people at his institution go over all the material before that appointment.

Next day, he calls mid-morning suggesting that it might be worthwhile to rethink our plan. My reaction could be, "Aw, oh, here we go again," but it's not; what I focus on immediately is his comment that he spoke with the surgeon (the one who does do pancreases) last night. So, he thought about me and my situation in the evening and made some phone calls. And, because I like him, I credit his flexibility and note that he is preoccupied somewhat with my problems. Oh, Jonathan!

What he suggests is that since it took the tumor seven and a half years to get to where it is, it would make sense that if it were removed, since there is no sign of anything else anywhere on the CT scans, it would likely take years before anything else is noted—and then medicines may be even better. So surgery seems like a reasonable approach at this time, but he will present all my material to the next meeting of the tumor board (quite some terminology for a group of cancer experts reviewing difficult or complex cases) and call me to let me know what they recommend.

So he calls on the day he promised and says that all agree that the cells here are identical with those of the original cancer and that the tumor board and Charlie Linker and the surgeons agree that the best way to proceed is surgery, so I'm out of his benevolent hands and back in the hands of the people I have no trust in. But the rationale sounds so right, it seems I have no choice. And all the right people agree. Out of the depths of despair, I arise and call the pancreas surgeon's assistant, who tells me that everyone has been conferring (you will notice that *everyone* does not include the main participant: me) and gives me an appointment for the following day at 12:30.

We are there early, of course; I'm asked to fill out the one page pain form, I check *no* at the first item (since I have no pain), and return the form to the receptionist in two seconds. When I return to my seat, the surgeon's assistant and someone she introduces as a trainee approach a family consisting of a mother and two young women to give them information; in that very open waiting area, they talk about what I consider rather personal information, about finances, for example. My favorite moment is when the sister who is not the patient starts to say something, the assistant, in her piercing loud voice says, "May I speak," as though the young woman has shown gross disrespect of her authority.

At about 12:50 we are brought into an examining room, this time with no hesitation about which chairs to sit on. At about 1:10 I leave the room and suggest to the person who brought us there that it's already 40 minutes past our appointment time. She mumbles something unintelligible and before I can say, "Huh?" she's gone and I begin to pace and for the next half hour Diana and I alternate pacing the corridor and the waiting area. It's now 1:40 and Diana, having ceased pacing, is fixing her appointment book and making phone calls. Except for an occasional stop back in the examining room to express disbelief at the hour and to swear a bit, I pace. At 1:55, my pacing is interrupted by the surgeon's assistant who bumps into me, greets me heartily, and apologizes when I comment that I've been waiting an hour and a half. She wonders whether the resident has been in to see me and then says that they are running late (could have fooled me) and that they will be in shortly. Fifteen minutes later, she approaches me in my now continuous pacing to say that the surgeon himself is right now on his way to see me. It's now 2:10. I have to admit that during my pacing I've seen the surgeon and a coterie of residents and medical students going into examining rooms, rushing into a room labeled *Residents' Room*, where they sit looking at computers and films on light boxes.

At 2:20, the assistant passes me and mentions that they are waiting for the material about the interventional endoscopy; I tell her that I have a copy and would be glad to let them see it. I make an error and say that I had given it to them last time I saw them; she points out that it was done after I saw them. I remember afterwards that it was to Dr. Rosenberg I had given it, but I guess these boys have not yet learned to share.

I'm still pacing at 2:35; I'm close to my examining room and a resident and medical student, walking toward the room, ask if I am Mr. Singer. I insist that they precede me into the room and we begin. They introduce themselves, and the resident, looking at papers in the folder he is carrying, asks me questions about pain (they are obsessed!), symptoms, other medical problems, etc., each of which I answer, commenting on occasion that the material is all in the folder. I explain to them that my irritation and stress is from having been kept waiting two hours and five minutes; their response is an apology and again the explanation that they are running late. "All the cases we see are as complex as yours and need attention," the resident says, and I respond that one ought to schedule with that in mind. With that, I drop the attitude.

The resident explains that since the tumor and lymph nodes that are affected are on the tail end of the pancreas, then that is the area of the pancreas that will be removed. If there are cancer cells in the blood vessels to the spleen, then the spleen will have to be removed. When I explain that I am feeling like the clones raised for body parts in a novel I just read, the medical student grins, but the resident says that they remove organs or pieces of organs only when there is a serious need for their removal (irony does not work well, it seems, in surgical quarters). He says also that they want me to see a cardiologist, because I am old and this is serious surgery. They leave—by now we are on the best of terms—saying that they will return shortly with the surgeon.

In he comes, followed by the resident and medical student. This time he is wearing a white coat, which to me does not bode well. Nevertheless, we (he and I) are all charm. But instead of setting a date for the surgery, he tells me that there is a nodule in my lung; therefore removing the pancreas material will leave me still vulnerable. I say this is the first time I've heard about this lung deal and he says that he wants to confer with *all* my doctors (I'm not sure if this is a dig at me) and that the resident will be in touch with me tomorrow. He says, "This time you'll have to wait at home," indicating, I expect, that my bitching about the two hour wait was inappropriate—gone is the grumpy, but kind hearted, editor of just a few weeks back. I respond with a smile that home is more pleasant than here. They ask that I wait in the waiting area until the assistant has arranged appointments for whatever has to be done next. We wait and finally it is the resident, not the assistant, who comes. He gives us his card, tells us he will call us tomorrow after everyone has conferred and if we don't hear from him by afternoon, we should call his beeper. He mentions that there seems to be a nodule in the splenic vein and that increases the probability of having to remove the spleen.

Well, there we go. Cancer in my lung and no more spleen! How will I vent my spleen now? (Forgive me for that, please. Sometimes I can't help myself.)

When we get home, there is already a phone message from the resident that the card he gave us has the wrong beeper number and he leaves the correct number. I e-mail Jonathan Rosenberg immediately about my lung and artery and he emails me back that in the artery there is a small blood clot; it does not seem like a cancer nodule and that he will speak with the appropriate people. At 10:30 the following morning he calls to say that he has spoken with everyone who needed to be dealt with and that he expects that we should now go ahead with the surgery. I ask about the lung and he says that it's been there for a long time and the size has not changed in years. It might, of course, be cancer and if it is this surgery will not be a cure, but I will get several years. His general demeanor suggests that he does not think it's cancer, but whatever he does think, he is responsive and empathic, and, for the moment, that's enough for me,

Early in the afternoon I beep the resident. Fifteen minutes later I beep him again. Ten minutes after that he calls and says that he has still to talk with Dr. Rosenberg and the radiologist. I tell him that I've spoken with Rosenberg, he asks what he says about the lung, I tell him, and he says that he will speak with him and get back to me within two hours. (So why ask me?) Anyway, he calls me back, tells me that everyone agrees, it's to be surgery: the tail of the pancreas and the spleen will be removed; and the pancreas surgeon's assistant will be calling me after she has set up appointments for me prior to the surgery.

And indeed she does: infectious diseases for inoculations (because the spleen provides some immunity), a cardiologist

185

(because I'm an old guy and the anesthesiologist ought to know what he's dealing with), a meeting with the pancreas surgeon (so we're both clear on what's to take place), and pre-op appointment (mostly discussion with an anesthesiologist). She makes all the appointments (after I tell her what's good for me) and e-mails me the information, all very efficient. It looks like the rest of this month is filling up with surgery-related activities.

I had asked that the surgery be scheduled on a Monday, because, if I'm to spend five days in the hospital, a weekend will be involved if the surgery is later than Monday. But, as you might have guessed, I am scheduled for a Wednesday, with all the anticipated effects of an understaffed weekend in the hospital.

First appointment is with the cardiologist; after a technician does weight, vital signs, and an EKG, the cardiologist introduces himself and takes us to an examining room. The whole area has clearly been redone very recently and very tastefully, red patterned carpeting, lots of glass (some of it etched with donors' names), and nice wooden furniture. The view (from the eleventh floor) is sensational. He is a very warm, pleasant, literate man (when I tell him that I feel like the clones used for body parts in a novel I just read, he is familiar with the author), who tries to read significant parts of my file as he talks to me. After lots of questions and some physical examination, he gives me the OK for the surgery (only a one percent chance of some heart catastrophe during surgery, and since others have a one half percent chance, I'm good with that).

The pancreas surgeon's assistant had set up the two appointments two hours apart, so we arrive at the designated area for inoculations an hour prior to the appointment time, with newspapers to read and knitting to do. Two hours later, despite entertaining distraction from conversations with others in the waiting area about their allergies, their pets, their new pocket TV's, I'm a crazy man. But when the doctor does approach us, he is so impeccably dressed (almost ruined by his white coat), so gracious, and so apologetic, I melt immediately. I'm easy. He says that since he has received no material about me, he is not sure why I am there (the assistant was very efficient setting up appointments, but not, apparently, in communicating referral issues). Fortunately I know and am able to tell him; he explains about the problems attendant on a splenectomy, arranges for someone to give me two shots, gets some printed material for me and for my personal physician and also a prescription for an antibiotic should I get an upper respiratory infection, and we are out of there. Maybe twenty minutes all told.

Two days later, we are in to see the surgeon. As the assistant had assured me by e-mail, we are seen exactly on time and the manner and attitude of both the resident and the surgeon are at least deferential. At our first meeting, the surgeon began, you will remember, by saying that he would remove the pancreas and I would be diabetic; this time, he says that his intention is to remove the tail portion of the pancreas (and the spleen, but only if it seems necessary) and that it is unlikely that I will be diabetic; that if it is possible to do the surgery laproscopically, I will very likely be discharged after four nights. The surgeon is all reassurance, very considerate, close to warm: the editor has returned. I guess that all my pacing and complaining at my last visit paid off. It doesn't always.

As we leave, at the bank of elevators, we bump into the assistant and I mention that the inoculation guy said that he had received no referral about me; she says that she faxed it to him three times and that, anyway, it is in my file on the computer.

Two days before my appointment with them, I get a recorded phone call from the Prepare Unit (can you believe *Prepare*?), saying that I will be meeting with a member of the anesthesiology team and that if I am more than fifteen minutes late the appointment will be rescheduled; no mention of consequences if *they* are more than fifteen minutes late. But the threat is given in as pleasant a voice as a record can yield and I do know how bothersome it is when patients are late and I suppose that their experience is that "Please be on time" is not enough.

The morning of the appointment, Diana has to be downtown at 10:30. I drive her, leave her, go to pick up gin that we are short on (I have priorities), and get to the hospital at 11:00. I sign in and at 11:30, fifteen minutes prior to the appointment time, they call me to register and sign some forms. That over, I wait a few minutes and am called to someone else to sign some other forms and to fill out a form about the drugs I take. Since in the recorded phone call they asked that I bring a list, I hand it over, and have very little else to fill out. I then return to the waiting area, and am called by a woman who wants to take my vital signs, draw blood (how many times need blood be drawn in relation to this upcoming procedure?), and do an EKG. I explain that an EKG was done six days ago; she says fine, that she will get a copy, she does whatever else she has to do, we discuss her corn-rowed braids, how long it took to get them done (five hours), and how much more comfortable they are in hot weather, and I return to the waiting area. A few minutes later I am called by a woman who introduces herself as a nurse practitioner, who asks me a few questions to confirm material in my file (one of the items being the list of medications I take that was sent over from the institution where my interventional endoscopy was done and which I hope matches the list that I have just handed in). She says, on her own, that I cannot meet the anesthesiologist, because who it will be will be decided by lottery after 5:00PM the evening before surgery, but she assures me that one will meet and talk with me prior to the surgery. I am then free to leave.

It certainly seems that anything that did get done could have gotten done in maybe three minutes prior to surgery. And why the plethora of paper? There are computers in front of everyone. And the ridiculous repetition of height, weight, list of medications! Certainly none of those things is going to change in so short a time. We are not Margo in *Lost Horizon*. But no discussion of anesthesia and pain, my favorite parts.

We get to the room where we assemble for surgeries at 6:30 AM, when it's cold, foggy, and very windy outside. I won't go through a big deal about the two hours prior to surgery—you've been through that with me before—but I'll sketch in just a few highlights. The gathering room is already crowded when we get there, so, after taking some information, they tell some of us us to go to a second room. As soon as we see groups of people being marched from the first to the elevator bank, we know for sure that we will be forgotten and there will be no surgery. As soon as that knowledge becomes certain for us, a man comes into the room, calls our names, and takes us up to the surgery area. Though this is a modern hospital, mostly slick, with hard edges, the feel is of fog hovering on the moors. I change into a hospital robe, get onto a gurney, and we, of course, hunker down and wait. When the anesthesiologist comes in and offers me a choice between an epidural and something I've never heard of, I explain that I have no information on which to base that choice. She tells me that if her parents were in my position, she would see to it that they would have an epidural. I respond that that is probably the better choice for me then, but I don't comment on the absurdity of expecting a choice from me based on nothing; heaven knows, Prissy wouldn't have made a fool of herself and Melanie would have had an easier time of it, had someone explained to them that an epidural would have been terrific. Her comments to me (perhaps shrieks is a better word) to put my head down, to curve my back indicate how bad and disobedient a boy I am being, so I try, but really have no idea how to comply.

And then I'm in the recovery room and my surgeon is talking to me. Are you ready for this? They did a laparoscopy and discovered that the tumor is not on the pancreas, nor in lymph nodes, but rather is wrapped around, entangled with the blood vessels that lie between the pancreas and the stomach, so . . . . they could not remove it. I won't bother you with my inner monologue consisting mostly of varieties of "Mother fucker!" but one might reflect for a moment that in my case, in surgery, my target is never achieved. All these incredibly expensive diagnostic tools and it's like going to a shaman!

Soon Diana joins me there (she has snuck in and they are about to kick her out) and a nurse tells us that I am ready to leave the recovery room, but there is still a person in my bed in the unit upstairs (My bed? If it's my bed, why is someone still in it and no doubt eating my porridge?) Two hours later (yes, two hours!) I am told that my bed is ready but they cannot find the nurse who is assigned to me. One hour after that, in my mind a waste now of three hours of my now-to-be-abbreviated life, they have found the nurse and I am on my way up.

At this point, I am not depressed—angry, perhaps, but not depressed, because the surgery turned out to have been a necessary diagnostic procedure (and was, therefore, not a complete waste), because the original plan was medicine and we're back to that, because the doctors tell me that my cancer is slow-growing and far from life-threatening, because I am seventy five years old and however long I live, these years are a gift, and somehow it is clear to me that, in whatever minor ways, I can begin to assume control over what is going on. And angry! Angry because, in a nut shell, I've wasted time, I'm going to feel like shit, as one does after major surgery, and this time, no doubt, it's all iatrogenic: if there hadn't been surgical intervention (that went nowhere) I wouldn't have to go through the difficulty of recovering from surgery, and for people my age recovery is long. When I greet Diana first in the recovery room by saying that I'm a goner, I don't mean that I'm afraid I'm going to die, but rather, "Whoops, here we go again."

Since I have once before gone over with you some of the problems that are simply part of being in the hospital, I will try to talk here only about things new or different to me this time. The televisions are the same; the food and its placement are the same; the nursing staff is more pleasant, empathic, funny (I guess *human* is the word) than last time; the lung scan people are better than last time (at least until I ask the technician if anything showed up and she says, "I'd be practicing medicine without a license if I tried to read these for you"); since I don't come onto the unit for three hours after I was scheduled to (i.e., three hours closer to clarity), I don't end up with the same problems I had with the pain medication last time; I make sure that the door to my room is never closed when I am by myself, so I am never left alone with my imaginative (psychotic?) flights of fancy.

On Friday, two days post-surgery, my surgeon tells me that he will not be in on Saturday, but will be around on Sunday. I leave the hospital on Tuesday, without having seen him since Friday. Far be it for me to take the moral high ground, but you've got to wonder. And we know he is around and functioning since the residents tell me often that they will discuss with him things I bring up with them and they do come back and tell me what he says; not an efficient communication system, but one that he clearly likes.

So now let's get to the crucial issue for my remaining in the hospital. On my second day post-surgery, I get very out of breath, with any, even mild, exertion. Having had this experience in the past, I know immediately what the problem is. I ask how much blood I lost during surgery and they tell me, "200 cc." I know also that during the six weeks prior to surgery, my intake of Procrit was less than once every two weeks, and that the most recent time I neglected to take iron with it. This combination causes serious anemia in me immediately. I ask for a blood test and, if the results are in the direction I predict, a blood transfusion.

Initially I was supposed to leave the hospital on Saturday, but with my breathing as it is, no way. Since very little goes on in the hospital weekends, and since they have me down for tests galore, it looks now like the earliest I will be discharged is late in the day. I won't bother you with a description of much of the weekend, except for the fact that a respiratory therapist comes every two hours all night for me to breathe something in to clear my lungs; even though I explain that that is not the source of the problem, that my lungs are dandy, I do what they ask. My daughter Ruthie sleeps over one night, and even though the company is nice, I feel a little bad that she too is awakened every two hours by my respiratory therapist.

A very pleasant Indian woman, from *Pulmonary* (no noun is used), comes to see me and explains that my problem could be pneumonia (even though I have no fever, nor other symptoms) or a pulmonary embolism, which presents problems in treatment because one is reluctant to use anti-coagulants to deal with the embolism, when surgery was only a few days ago. Since a no contrast CT scan is unlikely to be helpful diagnostically, how about a sonogram of my legs, to see if there are any embolisms to start with and then a lung scan which, if there are ambiguous results, can be bolstered by what is learned in the sonogram. I explain that that is very interesting, but what is going on is the anemia, and a transfusion would clear things up. This is followed up over the weekend with two or three other members of her department to explain why it is important that I go through the tests, which I agree to every time they come, but I also add that the problem is anemia.

Along with that, residents from my surgery team drop by to say that, in addition, it would be best to be evaluated by a cardiologist and have a test done where a tube is sent down the esophagus and an echocardiogram is done from that position. I respond that I will talk with a cardiologist, but that nobody is going to be shoving anything down my esophagus. I again talk about my anemia and finally Monday morning a lab person draws blood. Although everyone now agrees that I am anemic and will have a transfusion later in the day, appointments are made to have the possibility of a pulmonary embolism checked out. (Is this a good expenditure of personnel and money?) I'm taken to have the leg sonogram done (results are not surprisingly negative) and when I return, I am given the first of two units of blood. The shortness of breath is gone! But I'll go along with them and a lung scan is done ("I'd be practicing medicine without a license . . . . "). I come back, get the second unit of blood, and could now climb the Empire State Building (or is it Everest?). I go to sleep, expecting that I will be discharged first thing in the morning.

At 6:30 Tuesday morning, my team of residents comes into my room. Keep in mind, won't you, that they wake you up between 6:00 and 6:30 AM, spend five or ten minutes with you, and then breakfast gets served after 9:00 AM. Do they wonder what you do during those two and a half to three hours? A very attractive woman introduces herself as the new Chief Resident (it's the first of the month and they change monthly). She is expensively put together, but there is a quality of middle Barbara Stanwyck (*BF's Daughter*, *Executive Suite*), maybe Mercedes McCambridge in *Johnny Guitar*, in that she seems resolute, this is a woman who arranges to get her way, suggesting the quality too of a concentration camp commandant in anti-Nazi WWII movies.

She says that I will stay in the hospital until the cardiac study is done. I explain again that I will be glad to talk to and be examined by a cardiologist, but that I will not have echocardiogram apparatuses shoved down my esophagus, and that I will be home today for lunch. I then ask, since the symptoms have gone away with the blood transfusion, what the concern is that they clearly want to keep me here longer. She says that off oxygen (I am still on oxygen), my oxygen saturation (the little gizmo they put on your finger) will go way down. I tell her that that is a puzzling statement, since they've never allowed me off oxygen and, therefore, cannot reasonably predict what will happen to my oxygen saturation numbers and, with that, I remove the oxygen tube from my face and hurl it undramatically across the bed (Well, OK. The gesture is dramatic, but the hurl itself is understated—it's a drop rather than a hurl). As she gazes at me as though I'm Charlie Manson, I suggest she come back in an hour or so to check the saturation. She says some ritualized thing about talking with the surgeon, states that she will be back by 9:30 (I never see her again) and starts to leave. She turns around and asks, "Where do you live?" I tell her, and she says, "Well, that's not too far," and leaves. Within an hour, my oxygen saturation, off oxygen, is 96.

The rest of the morning is torture: I've agreed to see the cardiologist, apparently there is nothing else they want to shove at or down me, so we wait and see nobody except the nurses who have to do their two-hourly vital signs, and the food personnel who bring me breakfast, placed always irrationally so that I cannot reach it without a struggle and who come to ask, six days after I am admitted whether I like the food, do I have food preferences, allergies, an appetite. I respond as though these are reasonable questions at this moment in my hospitalization. And then there are numerous threats on my part that I will be walking out of the hospital if they have not made sure that the cardiologist and I finish up in time so that I can have lunch at home.

And there she is: it's 11:45 and in comes the cardiologist, an attractive, energetic woman, joking with me from the beginning, and explaining that this consult is my surgery team's idea, not hers (nothing in my behavior, I am sure, has provoked this comment), but that she will check things out and let us all know how my heart is doing. While she is stethoscoping me, another youngish woman comes in, they look at each other and fall into each other's arms, with a good deal of laughter. It seems that this second woman is in *pulmonary*, they knew each other well in their residencies, and I can be only proud to have brought them together again. So now, the two of them, with two stethoscopes, are examining me and finding no problems to account for the no problems I am experiencing: one in front of me, one in back of me, then they switch, and despite the balletic quality and the good feelings from this reunion, they find nothing and tell me that I am about to be discharged. By this time, I'm wearing civvies. I am lying on my bed and a wonderful, humane nurse practitioner, the person who seems to have taken me on alone to expedite my discharge is removing my staples. The procedure is again grim, but less grim than in the past, and this time, I know it will end.

Now I'm sitting in the hallway, on a chair the staff uses while entering notes into the computer. My nurse for the day—the very one on whose account I was admitted an hour late six days ago because they couldn't find her—approaches and indicates that I should get into my room, for vital signs to be taken. I enter, sit where I'm told, and she puts the thing on my finger to measure oxygen saturation. Alas, it goes up only to 85. She tells me that what I will have to do is walk up and down the hallway a few times, so that it will rise, and I explain that I will do no such thing, that I am to be discharged and I will worry about the number. She leaves the room and returns with another woman whom she introduces as the charge nurse (I suppose I am to yield to her greater authority). I nicely ask what she wants, and, before she finishes her sentence, I point to the reading on the machine which, now that I have engaged in some activity and speech, reads 96, I am told to go to the nurses' station where a young man holds a wheelchair for me to sit on, he then pushes me down to the main hospital entrance, where Diana is waiting to drive me home.

Let me try to put this into some monetary perspective. My last three days in the hospital were an expensive waste. Nothing really was accomplished by keeping me in the hospital until Tuesday instead of discharging me on Saturday, except to know that the problems that I said were not problems were indeed not problems. Aside from the cost of the various tests and consultations and therapists and medications, the daily rate for the room at this hospital is more than $4000 a day. Over three days, with the other charges, I would estimate that those three days cost Medicare and my secondary insurer around $18,000, which I understand from reading the paper they cannot well afford.

About a week after dischage, I get a call from someone at the Center for Interventional Endoscopy: she wants to know how I'm doing. I chuckle, she says she knows it's been quite a while since my procedure there, I say that that is not what I am laughing about, but rather that their pin-pointing where the tumor was was a bit off and I explain. She apologizes, says she will talk with the doctor, and he will surely call me. Although he never calls, I get a form-letter from him a couple of weeks later, saying that since I was a patient in their facility, surely I would like to contribute money to enable them to continue their work. In fact, I surely would not.

Two weeks after leaving the hospital I have an appointment with Jonathan Rosenberg. When he came to see me in the hospital, he told me when he'd be going on vacation. So I know that this appointment was set up just prior to his leaving; I am not surprised that he is quite late for the appointment, rushing to see a bunch of patients before he leaves, and he does get some points when his assistant comes in, introduces herself, explains why he is late, and does a number on how much Ruthie resembles both Diana.and me—although, of course, she and Diana are not blood relatives.

Jonathan arrives; he examines me some, looks at my surgery scar, and says that it is not healed enough to begin Avastin for a while, maybe in a week or two. He wants me to have a CT scan of the chest (no need for contrast) and an MRI of the abdomen and pelvis as baselines, and that someone in his office will contact me to set up the appointments. He wants me to have blood tests done today and we get that done immediately after we leave his office. He is very straight during the interview, listing possible dreadful side effects from Avastin, and explaining why for the moment, of the drugs available, it is the most appropriate way to go. In a nutshell, the drug attempts to cut off blood supply to the cancer cells. Probabilities of success are not great, but they do exist and I would rather not die for a while.

Next day, early afternoon, someone from his office calls. My creatinine is over 2.0, around where it's been since the removal of the kidney, and they would like to see if they can get it down by my drinking eight eight ounce glasses of water a day, and then having the creatinine tested again in a week. So, I'm into it. I have been engaged into doing something perhaps productive for me. No matter how water-logged, no matter how drowning I feel, no matter how many times I get up during the night to urinate, they've got *me* doing something for *me*. I mean I'm not yet over that iffy, tentative feeling from surgery and I feel I risk nausea every time I hold a glass of water in my hand, but I, at least, am trying to get my one kidney to kick in a bit more.

I am my own agent. However loathsome the process, I may be producing more efficient kidney function.

So now it's four weeks since the surgery and I have an appointment to see the surgeon for what I like to think of as the kiss-off meeting. I am, of course, early for the 11:30 appointment, I fill out the pain sheet quickly, sit idly (there are no magazines in this waiting room and I've forgotten a book; the only reading material is a stack of brochures encouraging volunteerism at the hospital, and, at about noon, someone calls out, "Paul Robert" (I have no idea what sense to make of this) and takes me to an examining room, where there are two magazines and where I wait thirty five minutes before a resident and medical student come in. The resident does the usual: "How are you feeling?" "Are you gaining or losing weight? ("I'm losing, trying to take advantage of the weight I lost in the hospital to get down to where I should be." "I want you to gain weight.". "Sorry, 'you can't always get what you want!'"), "Let's take a look at the scar," followed by how good it looks (to me, of course, it's almost unbearably gross and unsightly) and how dandy it's healing. After some good-natured banter, he says that he and the medical student will leave and bring the surgeon back, and out they go. It's all very easy, very comfortable.

A few minutes later they return with the surgeon, who comments that I look good, who is very personable, and who is lavish in his optimism about my prospects for the future: phrases issue like slow growing, non-invasive, small, many years ahead, ripe old age—and, of course, the more he says, the more lovable he becomes. He also seems very happy to be saying these things. I ask how much longer it is likely going to continue to hurt, and he says it generally lasts a couple of months, though with some people he remembers it lasting more than a year. He adds that a heating pad eases the pain and may also help the healing. (He's waited until now to tell me this? I had dope dripping into me all the time I was in the hospital from which I was discharged with a prescription for, to me, very heavy pain killers and when I ran out of them, the pain now considerably reduced, I grin and bear it for weeks—and all I needed these more than four weeks was a heating pad?) And then, no need to see him any more, healing very well, and an expectation that my oncologist and I will work out a way to keep things at least stable, and well-felt handshakes all around.

A day or two after the surgery, a resident has told me that the surgeon had taken excellent digital photographs of my tumor. What a prospect! Photos of my own insides in technicolor, my own tumor; not a frequently available opportunity. Vastly more real than an X-ray, a CT scan, an MRI, or a sonogram. Well, I have to have copies. So the last time I see the surgeon in the hospital, I ask him if he might e-mail me the pictures. Though taken somewhat aback and questioning the purpose ("I don't know why anyone who doesn't know what these things are would want to see them"), he agrees to send them. No pictures come. Home, a week later, I e-mail him, asking again that he send them. No response. Now, in the meeting I just described, I remind him, he says he will do it that afternoon; however, nothing comes. A week later, I e-mail him again to remind him, but no response. I suppose he agrees with me in person, in order to avoid any interpersonal unpleasantness, but clearly something about my having the pictures doesn't sit right with him. Perhaps he just doesn't want to take the time, without it bringing in money for the U and for him, but my feeling is that he is suspicious of my motives, though I can't imagine what arcane, dreadful plans he might think I have.

I allow my fantasies about the surgeon's withholding to flourish and then, exactly seven weeks after my discharge from the hospital, I get an email from him with my cancer photo. My paranoia is blissfully shot to hell, I love my surgeon now, and I have my picture that includes one side of my stomach. What do we learn from this? Wait seven weeks before making judgments.

And I keep doing the water thing, and it turns out that in about a week and a half it stops being loathsome, it stops making me sick to my stomach, and I learn to time it so I wake up to urinate only twice at night—a frequency I can handle. So I'm into it. The problem is that my creatinine decreases only negligibly, if at all. But still, keeping myself hydrated, as they say, (a state invariably lauded by those in the know) is a good thing and I might as well continue.

So, after a couple of weeks, it's time to start the Avastin. I am directed to the Infusion Center, two floors up from Rosenberg's office. I go to the reception desk, the woman there checks me in, and asks me to follow her to the waiting area. On the way to the waiting area, we pass or notice three large rooms, each with six chairs on which people are being "infused." The look is that of *Coma,* except the patients are not suspended, but more or less lying on Naugahyde LazyBoy-like chairs, many with relatives in attendance, but mostly silent, with eyes closed. Strange that to get to the waiting area you pass the *infusion rooms*, brightly lit and with windowed walls, all designed perhaps by a maniac. We sit for a short while. A middle-aged woman calls my name and we follow her as she describes laughingly her problems finding a chair for me, but she is successful in her mission and I take a seat.

The strangely shaped room, narrower than makes sense and with few right angles (homage perhaps to *The Cabinet of Dr. Caligari*, the shape of the room being, however, the only example of German expressionism), has five other infusees, four of whom have people with them, so the path nurses take to tend to their patients is hazardous indeed, and the wheeled legs of office chairs that the relatives sit on frequently trip the nurses trying to get through. There is no chair for Diana who hustles one up from the corridor outside, but my nurse brings her another and, laughing, says that the backless one that Diana brought is for nurses to do their work.

The nurse then wraps my arm in hot towels to bring out veins and make the IV easier. She leaves the room and returns in a few minutes, removes the towels, and says that they cannot proceed until they get information that insurance will pay for this, since the drug has not yet been officially approved by the FDA for my kind of cancer. She leaves and soon returns to conduct me to the office of a man who must be in charge of finances. He explains the issues: the drug is very expensive, if Medicare won't cover it, the drug company itself will negotiate with Medicare and, if they are not successful and I have to pay, will reimburse me. With this knowledge, I return to my chair, a woman brings in releases that I have to sign (one of them indicating that the cost of each treatment is $9,667—gulp!), I sign, she leaves, and my arm gets wrapped again for real.

I had been told that the first infusion will last ninety minutes and that subsequent ones will be a half hour. The nurse now informs me that the pharmacy has informed her that the protocol has changed and, that, once they get my doctor's permission, even the first infusion is only twenty minutes. And so it goes and we are out of there about a half hour after the infusion starts. A reduction in time from ninety to twenty minutes is a very good sign and I leave convinced that this drug will do whatever trick we need it for.

If we can tease out some success from this available drug, and there is no reason to suppose that we cannot, and I can feel that I am a collaborator in this success, well, what more can a person ask for? Having a diagnosis, having diagnoses, is no big deal for people my age. We swill pills like they are M and M's. The important issue is how well one feels, how one lives one's life, and how much control one feels. I've got it all in spades.

X

In which I find that now you have it, now you don't,
now you do

When I try to get up out of bed at 8:30 that Saturday morning in San Diego, I become aware that I cannot automatically sense where my right arm and leg are. I can move them if I look at them and concentrate. I hobble to the bathroom, thinking that this is nothing; not infrequently arms or legs are asleep, so why not both. Walking is difficult because I cannot quite feel my right leg, but I think the walk through and watch my leg as I do it, go slow, and don't fall. In the bathroom, although I can't pick objects up with my right hand, I am able to pick them up with my left hand and place them in the right. They will stay there so long as I look at them. It's hard though to look at a toothbrush or comb (the mirror, of course, confuses things) while using them, so objects repeatedly fall to the floor. Amused, I pick them up, but when Diana begins to pick them up, the amusement it is gone.

I manage to deny that this is anything like a stroke (Diana and I do not use a word for what is going on); I insist to myself that since the problems are on my right side, the left side of my brain would have to be involved and that would likely include speech centers and, although my speech is a bit loud and even perhaps slurred, I certainly can talk and thus, no stroke. But when Diana asks if I want to go to the Emergency Room, I say, "Yes;" playing it both ways, I am able both to deny and to take care of business. To my relief, she then suggests that I not shave and shower, activities that, although I've engaged in almost every morning of my adult life, seem unimaginable right now.

So Diana goes to confer with our hostess, Gail, a retired social worker and, therefore, pretty knowledgeable about the San Diego medical scene. Gail, professionally experienced in medical emergencies, knows how to act cool and rational, and she calls a physician friend for advice about which emergency room to take us to. He advises and off we go. But before we go, since we have a 1:30 flight back to SF, we have to pack; the idea is to go to the airport from the ER. (Packing is not quite so absurd as it sounds. We arrived at Gail's place the night before. We are in San Diego for my grandson's high school graduation and were staying at Julie's—Diana's daughter—but because it's been a long time since we saw Gail, we arranged to spend our last night with her and unpacked only what we needed for the evening.) I am careful and slow in my walk to the car and Diana gives me physical support. The drive is no more than fifteen minutes and I realize along the way that there is now tingling in my hand; with what seems to be sensation coming back; anxiety is somewhat allayed throughout the car.

At the emergency room, there are orange cones in front of the driveway. Even with anxiety allayed, Diana jumps out of the car and starts throwing the cones away from the driveway; she asks no questions, she just throws. Two security guards run out of the building, ask what she is doing (even though it is very obvious what she is doing), give Gail directions about what to do with her car, and instruct us to walk in, which we do, slowly and with much effort.

We schlepp to the window to register, give the receptionist the information she needs. She asks me to sign a form, I realize and tell her that I cannot write; on her suggestion I slowly, with a lot of thought, make an X, and sit, expecting a long wait. It seems like seconds after we are seated, my name is called, we go through a door into the ER itself where the triage nurse has us sit by a desk very near the door. She is an older woman, supportive, but brooking no nonsense, and she tells us to tell our friends and for us to know in the future that, in situations like this, you don't drive to the hospital, you call 911. (I cannot redo this morning; she means next time. Oh Christ!). She is a cross between Thelma Ritter and Estelle Getty, and reminds me of the supervising nurse, Agnes Bain, who was my boss when I was seventeen, working as a nurse's aid at the Boston State Hospital (why this job at that age is another long story); once she invited all of us under her supervision to a Christmas celebration at her house and, at the urging of many, sang *Danny Boy*, and, though unfamiliar to me, a Jewish boy with Eastern European parents, I understood immediately the flow of tears in the room.

But back to San Diego. I won't bore you with all the events, the tests, the questions during the six hours I spent in the ER. But, a few comments. Everyone I deal with is pleasant, respectful, attentive, reasonable, and adult and they treat me as though I too am a reasonably intelligent adult. After I have been there about an hour, all numbness is gone, soon a resident comes in with a coated aspirin for me, they do a CT scan of my head, and many conversations with nurses, residents, and attendings. During the six hours I'm there, Gail is in the waiting room: they allow only one person with the patient and, since that's Diana, Gail cannot stay with us. She does, however, come into our area every so often to see how things are going and she does have at least one visitor in the waiting room (the fellow who told her on the phone to bring us to this ER), but none of that is distraction enough for a six hour wait. We urge her to go home and we promise to call, but she is stalwart and true and will not leave her post.

At first, the staff expects to keep me overnight, but as the hours pass, the symptoms dissipate, and all tests negative, their plan moves to 1) I will stay in San Diego overnight, to 2) I can fly to San Francisco, but will go directly to a hospital from the airport, to 3) I can go home. Their impression is that I'd had a TIA (transitory ischemic accident), that a blood vessel has cleared and repaired itself from a blockage caused by the flaking off of plaque in a blood vessel and that, now on aspirins, the likelihood of recurrence is low. They want me, however, to see a stroke maven in San Francisco to follow up.

Lucky son of a bitch! No stroke, no damage, no extra stay in San Diego, and I am treated nicely the six hours I am there. So we leave at three o'clock with the name of a stroke man here in San Francisco. Our plane was to leave originally at 1:30 and Diana had called to shift it to 5:00. There is a charge of $40 each to make the change, but if we send the airline proof of this medical emergency, they will deduct the $40; we get the proof, fax it to the airline during the week, and the $80 ($40 each) is refunded.

So Saturday evening we are back in SF, call my kids, let them know what happened, and invite them to come over Sunday afternoon (this is to prove to them that I am in good shape, so they will not keep asking). They come over and spend a couple of hours with us. I notice before they leave that my right arm is somewhat atingle and peculiarly numbish, but I have no idea when it began and I tell them nothing. So there goes the TIA, there goes the no damage; it was a tease. In fact, I have had a stroke, one I can live with; I can do anything with my arm, it just feels a little funny. I decide, since this problem is milder than it had been the day before and since I have no idea how long it has been present, that I will not go to an ER (forget the instructions of the triage nurse!), that I will try to see my primary physician the following day and that I will try to get an appointment with the stroke guy as soon as they have an opening.

I am very successful with my primary physician: he will be able to see me at noon. With the stroke guy, it's a whole different universe. Not only is there no possibility of an appointment for six weeks, but they want me to fax them all the material (12 pages) that the ER gave me on Saturday. I fax the material, but notice that sometimes more than one page at a time slips through. When I finish I call the office to find out which pages got through; there is a problem since the 12 pages are really three separate groups of 4 pages, each numbered one to four. The secretary has trouble understanding what I am asking for to begin with, and the repetitions of numbers seem completely to floor her. As we continue to work on the numbers, we become a bit friendlier and she mentions, as though I now deserve to know, that there are times available within the six weeks, but the doctor is on stand-by during those times and if person with a stroke comes into the ER, he will have to leave me and go there. Having no numbers with which to analyze the probability of such an occurrence, I say nothing more than "Uh-huh," we finish the counting, I fax her the missing pages (very carefully), even though I expect never to use them since she seems convinced that the maven's on-call status is a very bad idea for me, and probably nixes the likelihood of an appointment.

I see my personal physician at noon. He seems comfortable with my situation, tells me to continue with the aspirin that was started in San Diego and, just to be safe, puts me on a small dose of Lipitor; even though my cholesterol is not very high, there is evidence, he says, to suggest that the probability of a stroke is reduced with Lipitor. I leave his office considerably reassured, feeling in control, and having no need to see the stroke guy.

The following morning at 7:45, I am awaked by a phone call from someone who introduces herself as Sonia. When she tells me that the doctor will have time to see me a week from tomorrow, I realize who she is. She has perhaps assumed a greater friendliness than I had and must have thought that if she is awake, I too must be awake. She is a bit apprehensive because it will be one of his on-call times, but says that he feels it is the right thing to do. Two days prior to the appointment I am to have an MRI of my brain. OK! There goes my yesterday's freedom, because I simply cannot deny this hard won appointment.

The MRI is late afternoon on a Monday. I go to the hospital, whose entrance is at its northern end. The MRI place is on a sub-basement floor at the southern end of the hospital, literally a city block away. I trudge the surprisingly long corridor (a city block is, after all, a city block), but when I arrive, there is no one in the reception area. I leave the waiting area, enter the bowels of the MRI area, and find a woman who seems to be official and is doing some work there. She notices me, calls me by name, apologizes that there is nobody in the waiting area, and guides me back there. I sit and she brings me some forms to fill out;

she says, quite apologetically, in case I have something planned for later, that she wanted me to know beforehand that something came up and I will have a half hour wait. Against my better judgment, I hear myself saying that that is unacceptable, that if I had a responsibility to be on time, so do they, etc. Fortunately I am saying all this quietly, my tone expressing no anger, but still! What am I doing to this woman who has been only kind to me, who, rather than surprise me with the wait, lays her cards on the table? Feeling like an ass, I finally stop, *she* apologizes and goes away. She returns in a few moments to say that if I parked in the hospital garage, she will validate my ticket because of the inconvenience. In the nicest way I can muster, I thank her, but say that I have parked on the street (my parking karma is way up there). I've behaved badly here, and still I have to reject her graciousness to make amends; would that I had parked in the garage.

As promised, thirty minutes after the appointed time, they call me in for the MRI. The procedure itself is uneventful and the technician goes out of his way to make up for the horrendous noise (perhaps brain MRI's are by their nature louder than others) with acts of kindness and pleasantness (or perhaps the woman who greeted me has warned him). Forty minutes after we start it's over and I am out of there, to walk the full city block to the hospital exit.

Two days later, we're at the stroke maven's office. As is standard, the first person to deal with us is a resident, this time a psychiatric resident, less than a month into her residency which begins apparently with some neurology experience. When she learns that I am a psychologist she tells me that she *just loves* psychology, and the interview and examination continue. I learn that she is from Boston and we exchange positive comments about the city where I too grew up. She learns that aside from some funny feelings (or lack of feelings) in my right arm, I have no neurological symptoms. She finishes the exam, says that she is going to get the maven and will be right back with him. They enter and she, nervously, does a little speech about me and what she learned. He seems delighted with her performance and then re-does the entire interview and examination with me. He too, it turns out grew up in Boston, and the "small world" comments proliferate; as a matter of fact, he says, it's amazing how much of the hospital's professional staff is from Boston.

He is a very energetic young man, with little reticence. There is a tennis player's quality about him, athletic looking, strong and quick responses, always making points. There are no shades of gray. He says that although the radiologist missed it, there is definitely damage on the MRI from my stroke and he points to a tiny white area. (In his formal report, however, he states: " . . . MRI scan reveals *a suggestion* of an ischemic lesion. This is not identified on diffusion weighted imaging." So much for definitely!). He goes on to tell me that this stroke is related to hypertension and that that fits well with my labile blood pressure and that I must have been under a lot of stress in San Diego; that I need to exercise (walk a half hour, four times a week) and learn techniques to handle stress without my blood pressure going up—that since I am, after all, a psychologist, I surely can discover such techniques and use them. The psychology I know has to do essentially with Freud; I've heard about bio-feedback, etc., but know nothing about that stuff. Freud will not help me with the lability of my blood pressure, but I smile and nod, and that's that. He says there's no need for me to see him again, because he will only tell me again the same things he told me today.

On the way out, I thank the secretary for putting everything together; she says that I needn't thank her, but that in a few weeks I will get a rating form from the hospital and it would be very nice if I rate this experience high.

So, I take my walks almost four times a week (my legs hurt from my intermittent claudication—but I do it), I take the aspirin, have increased the beta blockers, take my blood pressure now and then, mostly feel good and in control. Then I become concerned that I don't really know where in my brain the damage took place. So I call the secretary to ask that she fax me a copy of the maven's report and the one from the radiologist about the MRI. It seems I don't learn. I'm still expecting that if I make a reasonable request, I'll get what I want. Not so easy! She says that it will cost $25 for each. In the last 10 years I have been faxed many reports and never had to pay for them. And in this case, I referred myself for the neurological evaluation; one would think that a report would be part of the deal. I know by now that for some, doctors do official things only to or for other doctors; but that would not explain a $25 charge. I thank her for the information, ask her to send me whatever may be available at no cost, and immediately call my liaison to urologic-oncology, just to be able to tell somebody in the business about this latest development. She says that she will take a stab for me and next thing I know, the radiologist's report has been faxed to me. Meanwhile the liaison person calls me back to say that I can certainly get copies of the reports free from medical records at the hospital, a hospital different from the one where urologic-oncology is, making an exchange of records far from automatic.

XI

*In which I host another opening and am finally freed
from the tyranny of inpatient units and delusions*

OK. So after a year and a half on Avastin, the profusion of protein in my urine (a thought too weird and too generating of unpleasant fantasies for me to entertain for long) and increased creatinine in my blood suggest strongly that the drug isn't so terrific for my one remaining, lonely, seventy seven year old kidney. Since on a good day the kidney is far from 100%, we can't allow it more trauma, so we have to stop the Avastin. And with that, adios to my two life-saving drugs—Gleevec and Avastin.

There's not much else available to treat my renal cell carcinoma (that will not damage my kidney further), so we defer once again to the surgeons, hoping that a year and a half's worth of Avastin, which we are pretty sure has at least retarded the growth of my cancer, might have changed its form in some way that will now allow its surgical removal. My extraordinary nurse practitioner, Maryanne (who knows everything, dresses fabulously, worries about me, calls patients from the office after hours, talks to me like I am an intelligent adult, gets the jokes, and touches me when she talks) and my wonderful oncologist, Andrea (who has been here only about a year and who took a few months off to have and to care for her baby, who can quote the literature on a dime, whose very sweet disposition and gentle manner guarantee that she really gives a damn, and who gives off a sense of reciprocity) both are clearly very happy with the possibilities, and they become my sponsors. There is much back and forth emailing, the surgeons are sent whatever scans and write-ups are available and—surprise! surprise!—they send back word that with new techniques (such as *RFA*, radio frequency ablation, and *cyber-knife*—yes, honest to God, *cyber-knife*, as though the namers of these things have no imagination or they are stuck in some kind of sci-fi fantasy) they are quite sure that they can get the cancer out. My "sponsors" are delighted and they prod me into their joy. They, of course, will not be left with scars, pain, or hospital anecdotes, but there is the possibility for me of success here, of getting rid of this goddamn cancer. Appointments are arranged and I go to see the surgeons.

We wait, as usual, in an examining room for what I, as usual, consider an unreasonable amount of time and then, as usual, I begin to pace the hallway. I am approached by a tall, nice looking young man, with shaved head, white coat and black pants; he asks if he can help me and, when I explain my situation, he introduces himself as a surgeon who works with the man with whom I have the appointment (that is, the one who did the surgery two years ago), asks that we join him in an office, and almost immediately the main, senior guy shows up. They are very positive that the job will be done: they do not say, "Slam dunk," but that is certainly what they indicate. They talk about the MRI's, the Avastin, RFA (*cyber-knife* has apparently been dropped), as though answering my questions of why the results of surgery will be different this time from two years ago; and their affirmation is so strong, it feels as though they've answered and I too am more convinced.

I put the surgery off a few weeks, as though my control of the date is something more than a cheap thrill, and I use the time to develop an e-mail relationship with the younger surgeon. I need, and he offers, reassurance that only those organs that absolutely need to be tampered with during the surgery will be tampered with, and his expectation is that, at most, a piece of the pancreas may be removed, small enough that symptoms of diabetes will be unlikely, and nothing else. This works for me since, after the last surgery, word was (and the photograph I'd been sent seemed to confirm) that the tumor, intertwined with blood vessels, abutted, but did not invade the pancreas and that no other organs were involved. I push and push, he reassures and reassures, so what can I do but believe?

About a week before the surgery, I get a phone call saying that a third surgeon, whose name has been associated, in conversation with my oncology nurse practitioner, with RFA, would like me to come in to see him. Well, the more the merrier, so we set up an appointment and I go in. He's wearing a camels-hair jacket; every crease is meticulously pressed, every hair in place, he's neat, clean, and shiny. We exchange niceties, he says that RFA will not be used in this surgery (he does not explain why not; and didn't the idea of surgery come about, in large part, because of the magic of this new RFA? and didn't he become involved because of his expertise in that procedure?), that it will be a difficult surgery (maybe it would be easier if they were to use RFA!), lasting a long time, that recovery will be lengthy, that most certainly some of the pancreas will be removed and that therefore the spleen will have to be removed since an artery from the pancreas traverses the spleen (and he draws a picture as though I don't understand and the drawing will clarify things; it doesn't), that if his father, whom he loves very much and who is in his late eighties, were in my situation, he would advise against the surgery, but that he is ready to go ahead with mine. I shrug, tell him that without some pressing reasons I do not want these organs removed and that I will let them know if and when I do. And (I don't say this though) what does it mean that he will do the surgery that he would advise his father against; isn't there some ethical issue here?

The question for me now is: why don't I get answers from him—answers that satisfy, that make sense to me? I am not even remotely a person who simply goes along (as you surely have noted), and yet, when I leave his office, I don't know why everything has changed. The differences between before and after this interview are big indeed, and I've sat there metaphorically mouth agape, knowing that things are changing and I don't know why. I think I ask him to explain the shifts and, of course, he does respond to my requests, but what he responds with does not suffice to explain. It's as though we are speaking different languages each of us feeling that we understand the other, but when it's over, it strikes me that maybe there was a third, very similar language he was speaking and I missed, at the very least, nuance. It's bewildering to me; I don't feel that he's been obfuscating, but I just don't get what has happened. Perhaps, there is a need not to explain fully to people outside the club (i.e. the AMA) things that are perceived as medical issues. Or maybe, given his frame of reference, his world view (which I apparently don't share), he has explained it in full—and I just don't get it. It seems to me that my only options are to go along or to forget about the whole thing, but there is a cancer involved! What is a fellow to do?

At any rate, suddenly someone new seems to be in charge and the prospects are quite different from what I've been told by the people I used to think were in charge? So I quickly call my email buddy, who immediately reassures me that nothing is different, that the rather bleak picture I've just gotten is merely a function of how that surgeon presents information, that things will be just as he and I have spoken about in the past, that most certainly my spleen stays, and that, as a matter of fact, he will be *my surrogate* in the operating room: he will not allow *them* to do anything I don't want *them* to do. We then review my insistence that organs not affected must not be toyed with and we go our merry ways. I know that he is one of *them*, but he is a big fellow and his size reinforces his promise of protection, as do his good looks and easy manner, so I trust him and my own obvious moral high-ground, and I end up pretty sure that I'm OK. And I don't even question how this most junior person on the team has the power to set everything right. For me, power lies in the rightness of my position and in his general niceness. I am seventy seven years old and have learned nothing about how power gets distributed in this world!

A week before the surgery, I go in for the pre-op event; it's described in the material I get from the surgery people as an opportunity to meet the anesthesiologist, but, since I've been informed repeatedly over the years that the anesthesiologist is assigned by lottery the evening before the surgery, I recognize this to be someone's dream world and I expect nothing but a very brief interview, blood will be drawn, and an EKG will be done. The good news is that this time they find nothing wrong with me that might make me nuts again; the bad news is that the surgeon officially assigned the case is the pessimist who loves his father. I don't believe that loving his father is justification enough for usurping control of my situation; I know that in large institutions like this there are rosters and whoever is next takes the case. But I contracted with these other two guys and one would hope that that would mean something. I guess it doesn't. The customer is not always right. The best laid plans etc, and the whole thing is even more screwed up, because this guy would advise his father against the surgery (and he lets me know yet).

We get to the part where I'm supposed to sign forms, the most important of which (to me) is permission for the surgeon to do apparently whatever the hell he feels like doing while I am anesthetized. "Carpe diem," I think—and I refuse to sign. Now I am in control; like Ingrid Bergman in relation to Jose Ferrer, like Ben Kingsley to the whole British Empire, like all those resistance heroes and heroines in World War II movies in relation to the Nazis, I have defied *them* and made my stand for my freedom (and by extension, the free world). To my total mortification, they respond, "That's fine. You can work it out just prior to the surgery." Imagine if those fellows had said something like that to Ingrid; Joan of Arc's stature would simply have petered out. And what if Bogart had given the papers to Conrad Veidt: nobody would know the words to *As Time Goes By*.

I hurry home and immediately contact my e-mail guy. He e-mails me back that that's perfectly all right, that he will work up a document and bring it down to me right before the surgery and the ceremonial signing can take place then. You see: I have taken charge and everything now is hunky-dory, right? We have learned, however, that there is "many a slip 'twixt the cup and the lip," so, although I hate relying on things like luck, I am keeping my fingers crossed. I don't even ask myself or him at what point he is going to show this permission paper to his buddies in the OR.

One week later, I arrive, at that ungodly early hour, at the hospital, and am led with a group of my peers to that curtained situation upstairs to await the surgery. An IV is set up for me, I meet the anesthesiologist and explain to him that, in the past, opiates and other similar drugs cause me to be at least a little nuts, even with hallucinations (the results of this confession of mine are not a reduction of such drugs, but what seems like a ho-hum reaction from him and the addition of morphine to the list of things I'm allergic to while I'm in the hospital), my email surgeon shows up with a now acceptable permission form for me to sign, the surgeon who has now become the boss shows up to say, "Hi," and, next thing I know, I wake up in the recovery room.

My memory is foggy (we'll get to that later), but it seems to me that soon after I awaken, Diana and the surgeon are by my bed, and the surgeon is saying that the surgery lasted 9 1/2 hours, that they were able to remove the tumor entirely (YIPPEE! Wow! I am cancer free! They did it!), that a piece of my pancreas had to be removed and my spleen, of course, as well. Many things cross my very tentative mind and here are a few:

1. Holy shit!
2. If the surgery lasted 9 ½ hours, then I imagine that 9 ½ hours of anesthesia were required and what will that have done to my brain and my sanity.
3. All the energy I expended trying to retain my organs was for nothing; maybe I should have kept quiet; maybe being so open about wanting no organs out, pissed them off and they had to show me who really is boss.

4. The world is like "Dirty Pretty Things" and "Never Let Me Go;" organs *will* be harvested
5. Where the hell was my goddamn *surrogate*? Didn't the lying son of a bitch make the offer of surrogacy without my even asking? Traitor! Now it feels like they'll say anything to get me on the table.
6. Holy shit!

One might entertain the possibility of a silver lining even here (in addition to the historic, bell ringing, announcement that my cancer is gone) and I find that being spleen-less might carry two advantages. One is that, if you don't have a spleen, you should no longer be able to vent it and I have found that some people prefer people who do not show anger; my father, though, insisted that if you vent your spleen, for example, at clerks, you get more bang for your buck. OK. I'm ambivalent about calling this an advantage. The other advantage is that, without a spleen, you cannot get cancer of the spleen.

It is true that the surgeon told me that this was going to happen and it makes no sense for me to tell you that I didn't quite believe him, but it is alas the truth. We believe what we want to and, keep in mind, there were two guys telling me that my spleen would not be touched. Two to one; where would you bet? And I had my *surrogate* in there. What was to give me a clue about which of these people would have the most clout during surgery? It is enough to understand really that I, unconscious on the table, had no clout. Don't forget though that I told him that, except under the most demonstrably dire circumstances, I didn't expect my spleen to be removed and I even had my permission papers changed. So, what the hell, a promise gets broken.

Broken promises are one issue, but there is a more sensitive one here. Maybe there is complete justification for the removal of organs; maybe, but nobody articulated it for me in a way that made sense. The answers to my frequently asked question about why the removal are, "Well, we had to," or "The cancer invaded those organs." "We had to" communicates nothing and "the cancer invaded" is very hard for me to get with. A year and a half earlier, surgeons who operated on me and who saw and photographed the tumor said that it had invaded nothing. This was followed by a year and a half on Avastin, which was supposed to shrink the tumor and which we know from scans certainly did not allow it to grow. Invasion of organs, then, seems unlikely. The scans just prior to surgery, even with problems in perspective, seem (I'll allow maybe a bit of ambiguity) to reinforce the idea that nothing was invaded. So what is the story? Possibly, during the nine hours of surgery, the tumor simply could not be accessed for removal, so long as those organs were in the way. That sounds reasonable. So, if that's it, why not tell me? I don't know. I don't seriously think that these surgeons are really bad guys who arbitrarily remove organs from certain people on a list. I expect they had good reason, but they sure get funny and at least vague when I ask them. And it's conspiratorial: they all back each other up in the vagueness. Anyway, I am perplexed: is it that they don't take my questions, and, thus, me, seriously or do they feel that the truth is something that the patient need never know?

I don't remember being taken to my room, but I do remember, even in my foggy state, my delight at the very large, very slim flat-screen TV on the wall. The room seems to have been redone recently and it looks terrific, very (as the TV reflects) patient-oriented. It shouts, "All the conveniences of home." Although I never learn myself how to master it, the lighting can be varied many ways from the bed, and it all seems dandy. For that matter, I never master the phone: I know how to get an outside line, I know my home phone number, but it never works for me and I always have to get an employee to dial for me.

The next seven weeks are mostly a blur: there are large holes in my memory, nothing has sequence, I am frequently delusional and paranoid (more about that later), places and walls are fluid and insubstantial, cause and effect are mostly gone, changes in the location of the room, the hospital, and even city landmarks are frequent; my world, for this long moment, is built on sand and actual geography is irrelevant to my thinking. I have to outwit *them*, *them* being just about anyone I deal with besides Diana, Annie, and Ruthie, and sometimes, frankly, I worry about them also.

My hospitalization takes place over a seven week period: the surgery was on November 10 and I was discharged for good a couple of days before New Year's Eve. In the middle of those seven weeks, after about 2 weeks in the hospital, I was home for maybe two weeks that included Thanksgiving and I was back in the hospital for Christmas. I am unsure which of the events I remember took place during the first or second time in the hospital, but for our purposes right now, I don't think it makes any difference. I was quite a bit less nuts during the second hospitalization, but physically sicker, so it evens out.

A few days into my first hospital stay—I have no idea how many—just in case I don't notice that there is always, even during the night, a nursing staff person in my room, sitting and reading, ready to take care of anything I need (and this is no hallucination), Diana explains that the hospital has supplied a person to be with me all the time. I realize that this service is available to me either because I'm very sick (but then so are many people in the hospital; that's what hospitals are for) or I am totally nuts and need watching and protection (a more likely option, since that is not the case for most hospital residents, by which I mean patients, not doctors in training). I remember almost nothing between the recovery room and this statement of Diana's, but I figure that I must have engaged in some pretty wacko behavior. Maybe better not to know exactly.

Let me give you some examples of what happens to my perception and thinking. The TV occupies about a third of the wall opposite me in my room, and it seems to me that the wall and floor are hinged, so that the bottom third of the wall can become the floor, and the floor, then, the bottom third of the opposite wall, never mind the furniture. When that happens, I am standing precariously on a ledge made by the edge of the floor, now one third up the wall, and somehow, for reasons I cannot understand, what becomes the floor is just barely covered in water. Since the TV now rests on the floor, I am concerned about what harm the water will cause it. All this takes place so that the staff, situated behind walls and above ceilings can observe my reactions, test me out, and, in effect, cause me misery; it is them against me and they are in control (I might be nuts, but that sentiment surely is an accurate reflection of my situation).

It seems that nothing has boundaries. Day and night melt into each other. Numbers on the clock in the room tell me the hour, of course, but the issue of AM and PM is an irrelevancy. Although the window in my room should be giving me clues, I am unclear and mostly unconcerned about whether it's night or day; I can vouch for its being day only when visitors are around. When I'm awake I assume that it's day and personnel sets me straight me when I ask their help to make phone calls, for example, after midnight.

Good things too seem to happen. Jennifer Lopez has me for brunch, al fresco, outside her hillside house in Marin County. Whether or not Jennifer has such a house is moot; my idea is that to get there I merely walk out of my room and, with no regard for bodies of water nor bridges, there I am! And it is, as befits a diva, lovely, perhaps a bit understated, and very elegant. There are many details: her husband—not her actual husband—and his brother are there, the menu was specific but I've forgotten it, the mood is quiet, somewhat serious, though everyone is of good cheer, and they treat me naturally, like one of the family.

There is one door into my room, off the corridor, I notice, however, people coming in through any of the sides of the room, even the side with the window, thirteen floors above the ground. At times I feel that there is a patio outside the window which becomes a door. Now and then early morning staff meetings are held on the patio, but it's too dark out there for me to see who is attending. At times I know exactly where the door is, where the window is, where the bathroom is, and what is on the other side of the wall on which the TV hangs, but that knowledge is ephemeral and transient.

Of my three surgeons, one of them, the senior member of the group, the one who photographs my cancer, seems to have disappeared; no explanation. I simply don't see him any more. I am left with the fellow with the father and my e-mail buddy. At various points in my hospitalizations one of them tells me, early on, that, during the nine and a half hour surgery, I had a heart attack. Another tells me that I had two. I protest (why, I don't know) and he says, "No, no, it showed up on a blood test." Well, if they didn't notice it and they needed a blood test to tell them, I'm not too impressed, especially when they can't even agree about the number. During the second part of this hospitalization, I am told by several people, that I have fluid in one of my lungs; isn't that called pulmonary edema and isn't that a sign of heart failure? One day one of the doctors tells me that because of the heart problems, they are concerned about my blood pressure and they have put me on a new medication. I ask if the medication is a diuretic, he says yes, and I respond that, in the past (and he can check in my file), when I've been put on diuretics, there is consequence to my kidney (my creatinine goes up as does the protein in my urine); there is a slight acknowledgement that I've said something, But nothing more, and a few days later (probably because my blood pressure has not decreased—given my track record with these people, it simply cannot be because I objected), the medicine is withdrawn.

There is a youngish woman in to see me at least once a day. Although I might have been told what her function is relative to me, I don't remember. I get to think of her as my boss. She comes in a white coat, accompanied by her entourage of one, always the same one, asks me almost nothing, and what she says always sounds like an admonishment: "You've lost weight." "You have an infection," etc., like I've done something wrong. Her entourage, a young man, always smiling in a way that suggests that he is expecting a joke, is very likely a resident and she his attending. He says nothing, even when I address him directly. My destiny (in the hospital) seems to be entirely in her hands; whether I'm to be discharged, what medicines I am to take, what I'm given to eat—all these things are apparently hers to decide, and I don't even know what her title is. She comes to me knowing pretty much what the monitors and all the tests have indicated since I saw her last, the content of every conversation I've had with personnel that day, but seems completely uncurious about how I feel and what I think; it's as though she knows everything of consequence to her (and, of course, to me) beforehand. My experience is of no interest. She questions nothing; she conveys that her understanding, her knowledge is absolute; only *her* ideas are the truth. The only explanations offered about anything she tells me—and remember I'm quite nuts much of the time and retain very little, so a little explaining could help—is what my numbers indicate. She speaks very quietly, but that does not belie that she is something like God incarnate, for all practical purposes, omniscient and omnipotent in relation to me in the hospital. Bedside manner appears to be an irrelevant concept. Her beauty and mystery, her mute entourage, all add to the awe and wonder.

A few days after the surgery, I am very short of breath. I do anything at all, and I'm panting like after a marathon. It doesn't show up right away, because at first I'm moving very little. When it comes, I know from my previous hospitalizations (and I explain to anyone who comments or who looks nervous) that it's due to loss of blood during surgery and the inefficiency of my one kidney in producing erythropoietin and that combination results in anemia which is responsible for the shortness of breath. I get patronizing smiles, lectures about my heart attack(s), references to a pinpoint on my lung (no one believes it is a radioactive iodine pellet gone astray during my brachitherapy for prostate cancer some years ago, even though the doctor who did that procedure told me that that happened and I repeat that to everyone connected with my x-rays), examinations by cardiologist, lung people, many x-rays, visits by respiratory therapists (when they come every two hours during the night, I finally tell one never to return while I am sleeping!) who insist on my doing breathing tasks, no matter what I'm doing, whatever the time. Imagine how much money Medicare is paying for all these tests and consultations! I alone can be breaking that bank. Finally I am given a blood transfusion, my hemoglobin rises, my shortness of breath dissipates, but nothing gets rid of the heart and lung consultants nor the respiratory therapists (who even give me one of the blow-into apparatuses to take home).

One day, my e-mail buddy, my surrogate, comes to see me. He has been mostly cool, keeping his distance, still nice, friendly, and concerned, but you can feel the distance. He must be aware, of course, that during surgery he abdicated his role of surrogate. Perhaps he is afraid that I will confront him about his betrayal or that I will sue him for not adhering to the spirit of the consent form I signed (and he's probably thinking that if he is not around, I will forget about him and do nothing unpleasant). He is very excited now, like he's just witnessed an eighty yard touchdown, and he says, "I've been reading the literature and there's good evidence that when renal cell carcinoma metastasizes near the pancreas and it's removed with good margins, it doesn't return." (How might anybody do anything untoward to the bearer of this news?) He punches the air with his fist, falls into an armchair with glee, and the room is brighter with the contagion of his glee. I had heard these results before while weighing the idea of surgery, but having it affirmed, after the surgery, when the thing has been removed for sure, and knowing about my margins, and seeing his joy validates it all. And it's clear that this man, the relinquisher of his surrogacy, is now very happy, not only for his success, but for my future and for my well-being.

Nurses come by many times a day to give me pills and shots. They name the pills and tell me what they are for; with a few changes, they are supposed to be what I take normally, but a lot of what they name I've never heard of. I suppose that I am used to a particular brand name and the hospital might use different brands or generics, but for all I know they could be giving me arsenic or placebos. Of course, I question what is not familiar, they humor me a bit, treating me like a paranoid nut (which I am, though not in this area, and it's hard for them to discriminate). The shots are all new and they vary daily, maybe hourly, because they are summoned up to deal with the numbers on my monitors and tests and nobody seems to realize that changes as small as what is registered may not mean significance. And they do like to treat and I accept what they give me. I figure that, in the hospital, should problems arise, they will be noticed and attended to. At home, I can take eight or ten pills at a time; here, I gauge how sick I am by how few pills I can swallow at one time. Nursing people always also want to know whether I'm cold and need more blankets. I don't know whether they are really concerned about the temperature or is this a subtle reaction to immodesty on my part (i.e. my legs are showing and, despite my attempts to be covered, perhaps other parts as well).

During the second week of the hospitalization, I am told by residents (by which I mean doctors in training, not patients) who keep coming in to look at monitors (of which there are many) that my creatinine keeps rising and, if it continues to the point of kidney failure, they will dialyze me—not to worry yet, they suggest, because often a couple of dialyses enables the kidney to return to its prior level of functioning. Kidney failure! I don't have enough to be concerned about! I am frightened, of course, at the prospect of my one kidney failing, but somehow I know that should that happen, the dialysis will rectify the situation. But I do know too that if shit is going to happen, it's really going to come down, so there is no surprise when my creatinine reaches eight and a half (you may remember from much earlier in my story that *one* is normal) and the decision is made for dialysis. What I do not know is that, in order for the dialysis to take place, they need to put a port in my neck (does this location invoke Dracula to you?) that will stay there as the plumbing through which my blood will leave and re-enter my body for as long as I'm on dialysis. "Big deal," I hear you thinking. Well actually, "a big deal" it is. Here's the story.

A rather heavy-set, youngish woman comes into the room. Her hair-style, her attire, her speech, her attitude, her manner all suggest that she is a nursing assistant or, more likely, someone who cleans up the room, but she introduces herself as "a kidney doctor" (she does not even say *renologist* or *nephrologist*, whatever the hell the title might be) and says that rather than sending me down to the interventional radiologists where the procedure will be like surgery, she herself, here in the room, will affix the port and that will save me a lot of aggravation and trouble; that I need not worry, she has done this *hundreds* of times, and, worse case scenario, if she doesn't get it done (very unlikely, given those hundreds of times), I will be sent down to Interventional Radiology. She never looks at me and her responses to everything I say or ask are curt, conveying that it annoys her to have to listen to and register anything I might say. She promises to return soon and that everything will be done quickly. And return she does, this time with an older man, a renologist, who had been in to see me before and will remain during the procedure. Does this mean that in reality she has never done this before and he is here to instruct or, at least, supervise her? The procedure begins.

I am in bed; she is on the right side, he on the left. She anesthetizes the area she is about to work on and I feel no pain during the procedure. Very quickly, but very softly and quietly, he begins to make (across my body) "suggestions" and she indicates what she is trying (unsuccessfully) to do. She seems unrattled by his "suggestions" and by what appears to be her incompetence in the procedure (despite *hundreds* of previous successes). So far, not really confidence-inspiring and it goes on and on. I can see nothing of what she is doing because of the draping and because she is working on my neck, and I am grateful for that. His voice never rises and there is not so much as a wince in his manner; his is the zen of mentoring the fuck-up. Her voice never rises and she always sounds confident in what she is doing (maybe it is that delusional confidence that accounts for her statement about a hundred successes); hers is the arrogance of the fuck-up. I'm assuming that she is a resident (although "kidney doctor" does not really give us a clue), but one wonders how the hell she got this far. Finally after about a half-hour, but what seems like the entire afternoon, he "suggests" with great kindness to me and to her, that they stop, and he tells me that he will arrange for me to be sent down to the people in Interventional Radiology who do this all the time and there will be no problem. I tend to believe him (over her previous statement), but look at what he just allowed. She fixes up the wound that she herself just created on my neck and they leave.

Later in the afternoon, I am taken down to Interventional Radiology (the way things are communicated to me by nursing personnel on the unit, it's like the radiology people are doing me a big favor by having an opening to see me; isn't that what they are there for, isn't that how they make a living?). When I am wheeled in (I travel everywhere by guerney), I see that there are three or four young men and one young woman, all very attractive, all playful with each other, teasing and joking, (they seem not to have been doing anything anyway, so what was the fuss about getting an appointment?) and all solicitous to Diana (who has come down with me and not yet been asked to leave the room) and me. I remember the room as white and stainless steel, at least Buck Rogers. They are all very reassuring, making light of the aborted procedure upstairs, they explain about the procedure, and everyone (including us) seems comfortable. I am placed on a table that goes up and down, rotates, tilts, and maybe whistles Dixie, and Diana is asked to leave the room. My table (with me on it, of course) is positioned just so in relation to the complex x-ray paraphernalia that looms above me, one of the young men, wearing an excellent glen plaid suit, very well tailored, an especially beautiful, blue oxford cloth shirt, and a necktie, makes some additional minute adjustments, begins the procedure with a bit of patter, and, in perhaps two minutes, it is painlessly finished, without incident. I am now ready for dialysis. I can hardly wait.

So, the next day I'm wheeled to the dialysis area. There is no sound here. Aside from the silence and the mission of the place, there is no high tech, no chrome, here. It has the feel of *2001* or the beginning of *Alien*, but it completely lacks the look. Three or four people are sitting in what is supposed to pass for comfortable chairs, presumably hooked up to dialysis machines, facing a row of three desks, where two women are sitting, reading and writing in charts.

A young man approaches me; he has wild hair, speaks in an accent, looks untidy, and conveys an attitude that he is excited that there is someone new and neutral to talk to, that he wants to be my friend, and that he is the target of the women's anger. He says that this procedure will be easy on me, not to worry, although truly I have no anxiety about the procedure itself. He goes to one of the women at the desks, there is some whispering and their facial expressions are not pleasant, as though she is chastising him. He leaves (I am convinced that after trying to make me comfortable, he has been fired for being nice to patients), and silence again prevails. Finally one of the women, a motherly type, approaches me and asks if I am comfortable. I answer that I am and ask just how the procedure is going to work. She responds that the nurse who is going to take care of me will be here in just a few minutes and she will tell me. (Three things: if she is going to be here in a few minutes, why do I have an appointment for a time when she is out; second, since she is not here, would it kill this one to give me a little information; and third, why even bother with whether or not I am comfortable? I suppose that if I am not, she will tell me that when my nurse comes back, she will very likely make me comfortable.) She goes back to her desk, probably to formulate hexes for the scapegoat and for whoever else is on her list.

My nurse comes by, barely introduces herself, and, before I can ask her anything, moves ahead with the procedure, as though somebody else has already told me what to expect. At this point, it would be ridiculous to ask her anything about the procedure, since, in fact, the procedure is already happening. For the second dialysis, there's no need to get any information, because I've already had the experience. Suffice it to say that I am enormously grateful that, soon after the second dialysis, my creatinine returns to what has become normal for me, evidence that my kidney is back in operation, at its humble best. I guess that, for the moment and in this area, I'm willing to give up expecting civility, if they can return my kidney to its normal level of functioning. And that they sure did.

A couple of days later, most bodily functions back to normal, I'm ready to leave the hospital. It's been more than two weeks and I am very eager to get home. Everyone is happy: I didn't look so good even just a couple of days ago, and now, Phoenix-like, I'm looking good and ready to sail out. But once I get home (and manage to climb the ten stairs to our place), I realize how weak and debilitated I am and it gets worse. I am very wobbly: I need someone to watch me when I walk the hallway (I have avoided orders to walk enough in the hospital and I need the exercise and the practice). I have terrible diarrhea and no appetite. I know I should be eating, so I force myself to eat a quarter of a sandwich and that produces a new bout of diarrhea. I get more wobbly and feel weaker. It's a chore to get out of bed. We have a Thanksgiving dinner: our kids are around and I manage to be at the table for maybe fifteen minutes before I have to go back to bed. In infants, it's called "failure to thrive," and it's getting worse.

I have an appointment to see the surgeon about a week after I get home. It is a very difficult trip for me because I feel like shit, but Diana gets me to the hospital and we go up the elevator to the sixth floor. Off the elevator, I am so weak, so tired, so lacking in energy that I simply cannot walk to the reception are around the corner and down a short corridor. Diana hustles me a wheelchair from an open storage area and gets me to where we have to go. A nursing person suggests that we wait in the surgeon's office (they probably don't want other patients in the waiting area to see how lousy I look after surgery); they manipulate the chair into the office and the chair occupies the space so awkwardly that when the surgeon comes in, he makes a big number of going around me to his seat. He is very troubled and puzzled about my debilitation and, thinking out loud, he says, "We took out his right adrenal gland, but that can't account for this degree of fatigue." (Yes, it's about four weeks after the fact and I am just learning that I have lost a third organ. If this keeps going, what the hell is going to be left? And if I weren't feeling so lousy as I do right now when I am in to see this surgeon, I probably would never be informed that I am without my right adrenal gland.) I react with horror, muted, of course, because I have no energy, and his response to my questioning is like his response to my prior questions that, well, we had to remove it, the tumor was touching it. I say that I'm not comfortable with that notion until I can see some evidence, so (knowing that many photographs were taken during surgery—the senior surgeon, as I mentioned, is a camera bug), would he e-mail me a photograph. He says, "Sure," and a few days later I get a photograph of the tumor, already outside of my body, attached to nothing. So now missing are a kidney, a piece of pancreas, my spleen, and my left adrenal gland. Is there anything else that can be removed? But there is more to say about the office visit.

On reflection, it amazes me that he does not recommend re-hospitalization. I can't fucking walk! The diarrhea is terrible. I'm not eating. I feel like I'm just barely, and with great effort, hanging on. Clearly, Diana is understandably frightened. It is true that initially I might refuse hospitalization, but I am certainly not totally unaware of my debilitation and of Diana's terrible, though masked, fear. What can this Bozo be thinking? Maybe for a surgeon, if cutting isn't going to do the trick, there's no point in doing anything; why admit if there's to be no surgery?.

After about two weeks at home (that is, about a week after the above meeting), I agree, to Diana's relief (and that of my kids), that I have to go back to the hospital. She gets on the phone to speak with any of my doctors who will, for sure, admit me. None of the surgeons is around and she leaves them messages, but we don't hear from them. Surgery keeps them very busy. Finally she gets hold of the kidney man (the mentor during the aborted setting up of the port for the dialysis, the unruffled master) who says that he will meet us in the Emergency Room and get me admitted and we're off. Well, to say that we are "off" is beyond hyperbole. What we are is attempting to go. I inch down each of the ten stairs, holding on tightly to the banister, and begin the trek to the car, maybe fifteen feet away. I make it to the car, though I do question the possibility. As I wait for Diana to unlock the door (10 seconds perhaps) I shit my pants. I don't think that I "soil" my pants conveys anything close to what happened. The humiliation is unbearable. What do I do with my pants, my shoes, my soul, my dignity? I unbuckle my belt, unbutton and unzip my pants, and let them drop. I drop my underwear. I'm on the sidewalk, next to the car! I can't get back to the house; I won't make it. There seems to me to be shit everywhere. I don't know how Diana gets my shoes off; I can't possibly balance on one foot. She wipes off my legs with paper towels, I'm naked from the waist down on my street, I don't want to soil the car, I can't stop thinking, "It's come to this." Can't we erase this day? Can't I die or something?

I get into the car somehow, there are towels galore, paper and cloth, and, I don't remember getting there, but we are parked by the ER. Diana runs in and comes out with the kindest woman who ever lived, who pretends that shit is not an issue here, who covers me in a blanket, who gets me a wheelchair, and who brings me into the ER, treating me somehow as though I am an adult man who needs a little help right now. Sometimes even living people are worthy of beatification. We wait in the ER just a few minutes, and after a brief conversation on the phone, the receptionist tells us that she has just spoken with the kidney man and that we should go to the admitting area to be admitted. The kindest woman who ever lived relinquishes the wheel chair to the kindest man who ever lived; he wheels me to the admitting area, where I am briefly interviewed (nothing has changed since I was admitted last) and we wait for an eternity until the person about to be discharged from the unit I'm to go to is discharged, thus making a room available for me.

Finally I get up there and am brought into a double room at the very end (or perhaps you might say, "the very beginning"; half full, half empty) of the unit. The room is a long rectangle, but the beds, instead of being perpendicular to the long wall, are parallel to it, parallel to each other and perpendicular to the short walls, each at either end of the room, a curtain bisecting the room the long way, so that neither of the occupants can see each other, and when anyone wants to see him, they enter my part of the room and move the curtain to get over to his. Coming to the side of my bed, because of the narrowness of the room, one has to push into the curtain. There is good reason here for claustrophobia. At the end of the corridor, and therefore just outside our room, there is a door to the unit that opens automatically when approached and it is approached every time anyone enters or leaves the unit. There is a very quiet "whoosh" at the end of the closure. That and the narrowness of my setting, given the fragility of my ego at this time, are driving me even more bonkers. It's not that it's noisy; it's ghastly. I explain, ask to be moved when a room becomes available (I can't really tell them that I'm creeped out about the whoosh), and the head nurse sends me down a pair of ear plugs. I reject them, almost in tears, and within the hour I am moved to a single room, down the corridor some.

I remember almost nothing about the next couple of days, until I realize that I am in the ICU and that my hands are tied to the bed. I must be very sick and nuts again! I now have a feeding tube up my nose, a drain in my side again, and I am incontinent. I remember none of these insertions, nor the tying of my wrists. I would like to say that in this state staff needs a court order to do any of this against a patient's will and that in this country you can't force a person to take medicine that he/she doesn't want, but I don't know what the circumstances were in my case and, what the hell, in the long run, I'm still alive and functioning.

Diana tells me that the telephone wakes her at 2:00AM. The nurse explains that there has been a change in my "status," (well, why the hell else would the phone ring in the middle of the night in December, 2008), that I am in the ICU, and that she ought to come in. She drives to the hospital, expecting to find me close to death and there I am, a mask forcing oxygen covering my face, my expression like that of the guy in Munch's *Scream*, but alive! My take on the situation, at that time, is that we are at something like a cocktail party, surrounded by swells (like board members of The Opera, The Symphony, and The Ballet), all of us there to see some young doctors tout a new therapeutic device.

237

The device is applied to the face where it hardens and does its magic. It's applied onto my face (which I resent because I've not given permission), it begins to harden, and afraid it's going to hurt, I begin to pull at it; reality intrudes, hence the wrists get tied.

Here's the deal that I learn about later: I've had an infection (be careful of surgery and hospitals!) which they have smacked with antibiotics which have entirely screwed up my intestinal flora. Diarrhea is therefore rampant and that, combined with my not eating, has me mal-nourished and losing weight. In addition to everything else my thinking is weird, not quite so weird as a few weeks prior, but weird enough to keep me on guard, trust nothing, and develop strange explanations for things I perceive ambiguously. I seem also to have had a heart attack, so go know.

I am certain that my incontinence is as much psychological as it is physical. Certainly the diarrhea is torrential and sudden, but except for the one time waiting for the car door to open, it never happens those weeks that I am home between the two hospitalizations, nor after the second. Granted I wasn't as sick at home, but there is another component. This time, in the hospital, I am never sure where the bathroom is: its place, in my head, seems to keep changing. Also, I have to lug the pole with the drips into the bathroom with me and I'm never sure how it's going to fit. I don't have the energy. I don't call the nurses because, however quickly they come, it will be too late. The humiliation of a bed pan is too much; the grossness of being cleaned up is not an issue beforehand. So I let it go, and inform nursing personnel after the fact. It's seems like I am giving up.

I am told repeatedly that I have to eat more, that the ice cream that Diana brings me is not enough, and I concentrate on eating, a Herculean task, given my appetite, the kind and quality of food delivered to me, and the difficulty of reaching the trays once brought. Take the breakfasts, for instance: "orange juice" made of God knows what, scrambled eggs gelled into one mass, potatoes that are mashed, formed into cakes, then fried (I am willing to eat the meager crusts), and indescribable, extraordinarily weak, coffee. The tray is too high for me to eat from comfortably, because I can't sit all the way up in bed, and the coughing fits that ensue while I am trying to get this food down my throat convince me at each meal that if nobody comes to help me, I will choke, and nobody ever comes. I don't have the presence of mind to push the button for the nurse, but damn it, the cough is loud and terrible sounding, and can be heard, I am convinced, blocks away. I am cheered, however, that I survive each meal, and the reprimands (and they are reprimands!) that I am still not eating enough continue. They are force-feeding me, I have no appetite (except for ice cream), and they are criticizing me that I'm not eating enough. (I grew up with "People are starving in Europe.") I explain that when the diarrhea stops, when I am eating my regular diet, when I can eat seated at a table, when I'm feeling better, the weight will come back. But I don't quite believe myself and they certainly don't believe me. So the feeding tube stays in, and with it the constantly itchy nose, the surrender of control, and the mild to moderate paranoia.

So, I try to eat more. But they don't make it easy: the invariably dry chicken breasts (at home I eat only thighs and legs), the meat loaf, the pork loaf (my God!), the broccoli (surprisingly, not overcooked—as a matter of fact, it seems raw and hard to bite into—and it is the only thing that does not seem unhealthy; but it's not a favorite of mine), the pancakes, which to me look like sliced turkey (the syrup like gravy). The food isn't terrible, really; it's institutional food made up of things I usually don't eat, but most of all, I have no appetite and I am very uncomfortable. I eat the soup (which is usually excellent and thick) and nibble at the solid food; I'm trying, but not doing great.

Diana visits for hours, brings ice cream and good coffee. Ruthie, too, visits a lot and both she and Diana occasionally sleep the night in a chair by my bed. I never quite realize while I'm in the hospital that, in addition to wanting to keep me company, they are afraid that I am dying and that the fear is realistic. My surgeon, for example, the one who loves his father, comes by daily, often more than once and spends time with me. It almost seems personal. He looks very glum, says repeatedly that things had been going so well, why did they turn so bad? I later learn that he regrets removing the drain from my pancreas before I left the hospital, thinking now that the removal caused my infection. He appears to feel so bad about my condition (and my impending death, I think, in retrospect), that I end up reassuring him not to worry, that I will be fine. The presence of my six year old granddaughter keeps Annie away from the hospital; at one point, though I know we can smuggle Alexandra in, I decide that visiting me, feeling so lousy, attached to so much, would be too disturbing for her.

There is a continuous parade of people into my room: x-ray technicians (if you've never had a chest x-ray lying on a hospital bed, let me assure you that it is an experience like no other—the frame that holds the film is shoved under your back and, as you may recall, your back is not flat like the frame is, nor is it as cold), lab people wanting blood, respiratory therapists demanding that I do lung exercises, cardiologists, pulmonary people, nephrologists or renologists (it is surprising to me that there are so many kidney people in one institution), surgeons, residents of all persuasions, nurses who want me to walk, occupational therapists to teach me how to wash my face and brush my teeth (it's very similar to how I always wash my face and brush my teeth; but standing is very hard for me and sitting in front of the sink is a very awkward position, and practice under these circumstances does not make it better; I think their function really is not to teach, but to make sure I practice), physical therapists with their own axes to grind, nurses to play with the monitors when they malfunction and emit noxious noises (as they do frequently; it is surprising to me that some of the nurses who fix the problem say not a word to me—they walk into the room, over to my bed, play with buttons on the machine, the noise stops, and they leave), dietary people who bring food and those who want to know what I think of the food. And I am frequently taken off the floor for tests, scans, and repeats of tests and scans. All I want is to be left alone (with my wife and family) and I try (mostly unsuccessfully) to put everybody else and most requests off. I feel that it is sleep that I need, not walking needlessly up and down corridors, pushing or dragging my drips and their pole (holding onto the pole, though, does keep me from falling), or chatting with residents. Nobody asks how I feel, really; they think they know from the numbers they've gathered from my tests and the monitors or else it's not a concern of theirs. When I do say that I feel fine and just want to sleep, they ask why I don't watch television. Do *they* watch daytime TV? There are no premium channels here. So, why don't I walk? Because it's very hard for me (I have terrible trouble with balance and I am so goddamn weak) and I don't like having no destination. But I tell them that in a couple of

241

hours I'll get up and walk, but I'm lying. I'll walk when I get home.

In this context, I'd like you to know that during all these five weeks in the hospital, with all the professionals I deal with, none of them ever—not once—asks me what I did for a living, how I now spend my retirement time, do I like dark or milk chocolate, or any other questions that might reveal me as a person, instead of only as a patient. Isn't there some rhetoric about *the whole person*? On the other hand, the people who clean me up are extraordinarily nice to me. I am very apologetic for my incontinence and they treat it likes it's nothing. One of them even comments on my tattoo (obvious to many others). They sweet-talk me, they are reassuring, they never complain about this, from my point of view, onerous task, and never act as though I am putting them through anything untoward; they are more concerned about the condition of my skin, than about the unpleasantness of what they are doing.

After maybe two weeks back in the hospital, we begin to talk about the possibility of my leaving. The staff wants me to go into some rehab place, a skilled nursing facility, because they feel I need a good deal more nourishment through the feeding tube and that would probably require professional care to manage, I am still incontinent, and I am very weak: everything is a chore for me, on my feet I am off balance and wobbly, I do not like being out of bed, because of the infection that occurred last time they do not want to remove my drain yet and it needs to be cleaned daily, because a piece of the pancreas was removed diabetic testing needs to take place a few times a day. Their plans are countered by my wish to go home. Very simply, it's my feeling that at home I will flourish, nothing good will happen elsewhere.

The debate simmers. I am sympathetic with Diana's panic about my coming home—she tries to cover it from me, but alas, I'm a shrink and I can tell. From her point of view (and she doesn't really articulate it, but I know), she lacks the skills and energy to care for someone as sick (and incontinent) as I am, and she is as repulsed by the notion of having to clean out my drain daily as I am. My feeling is that at home I will not be so sick and that a rehab place will exacerbate whatever problems I have. Given this hospital experience, I know that in unfamiliar surroundings, with the mission of the staff being that I obey, that I function according to their point of view, not mine, that waves not be made, there will be nothing to enable me to flourish; no matter how long I stay there, I will be no better than the day I arrive. At home, I know where the bathrooms are, I will be eating better, and I insist that the care I will need is minimal. She thinks, reasonably, that my craziness is distorting my perception of my situation. I am, as it turns out, the only person on my side.

Everything is complicated by the fact that the Christmas season is upon us (Ho, ho, ho!), people are away, and it's hard to get information. When my surgeon (the one with the father) very sweetly tells me that the plans that he is involved in making are "for my own good," I realize that I can never do what this man suggests. When they say to an adult that something is "for his own good," watch out. This degree of condescension and arrogance (that someone feels he knows what is good for you better that you do) does not bode well; he wants to kill you (wasn't removing three of my organs enough for him?). Now, I know that he is not really trying to kill me: nobody is going to send him to prison on an attempted murder charge. But my subjective experience is that I have to beware of this man's concern.

His experience, I expect, is that here is an old guy, a bit loony these days, not really cognizant of the consequences of not being very careful, and someone has to take responsibility for his care. So he means well, but so, too, do other killers.

Finally the unit's discharge planner is back on duty. She, overly made-up and over-dressed, as though she's going to a party immediately after she leaves my room (and can't wait), tells me the names of three agencies that can take me during the next several days (this is the week between Christmas and New Years); she can't elaborate for me the differences among them and she can't give me any information that might be the basis for a decision. This woman does not match needs to resources, she matches discharges to openings. That's not what I need from her; I have a phone book and telephone, too. This helps my cause out a great deal, because I can now ask how we can even think of doing what she is suggesting when she clearly knows nothing. This back and forth goes on for a couple of days and finally I say, "What about a visiting nurse?" She says, "Oh, we can do that. (So why did she not start out with my going home with a visiting nurse as an option?) But I have to check to see whether your insurance will cover that." I'm on Medicare and I look to be of an age for Medicare. Shouldn't a person doing this kind of placement know what Medicare covers? It's not like it's a rarity to place someone who is on Medicare; I would suspect that a good percentage of people needing care of some sort when they leave the hospital is of an age that makes Medicare their primary insurer.

Of course, just as we expected, Medicare covers visiting nurses; everybody is now happy: Diana will have less on her shoulders, my surgeon will feel that my own good is being taken care of, and I have gotten to go home. But what if I, nutty as I am, hadn't thought of visiting nurses; I'd probably still be at some rehab place, like in *The Men*, in bed much of the time, trying to avoid doing what they ask of me, an invalid forever. Or they will have killed me, at least psychologically.

Now that a plan has been made, they decide that we need instruction; Diana is to learn how to prepare the tube feeding apparatus and I, since there are ten stairs to get up to our front door, have to practice doing stairs. Diana is so nervous about my going home and so willing (eager?) to rely on the home nurse, that she cannot really pay attention to the lesson she is getting. A physical therapist, whom I have never met before and whom I overhear telling someone that he is supposed to be at lunch right now, escorts me out of my room, opens a door off the hallway and, voila, a stairway. Remember those scenes in *Bullitt*? Slowly, with great effort, I walk up and down half a flight of stairs, he tells me how great I am doing (hell, I've been doing it seventy-seven years now) and I resent that the energy I'm using could have been saved for the stairs at home. He does not ask whether it hurts, nor how tired the practice has made me, but he lets me go quickly, he to go to lunch and I to bed.

Our discharge planner calls the visiting nurses agency the day before I am to be discharged and then Diana gets in touch with them to arrange when they will be at our house. A decision is made for the next day, late in the afternoon. Meanwhile someone from the company that deals with the supplies relating to the tube feeding arrives at our house the day before I get home, while Diana is doing her thing at the hospital, and leaves three boxes of cans of the food supplement I am to be fed and the mechanism that gets it into me automatically through the feeding tube.

The boxes of these canned goods are heavy and Diana cannot carry them into the house. She tries by phone to get the company to come back to bring the boxes into the house, but they do not show up. The boxes remain outside, despite the forecast of rain, and rain it does. The pole with the mechanism has been brought indoors.

Before we leave, a nurse wants to make sure that everything is in good order, so among other things she cleans out my drain and, in the process, accidentally (at least, I think, accidentally), gives the tube a jerk. I notice after that that, in certain positions, it hurts, as though the tube is rubbing against something inside me. I am not able to pinpoint the positions, but when it happens, if I move out of the position I am in, the pain usually stops. It's not terrible, so I can tolerate it and I don't say anything to anybody about it. I'm not sure why I am silent because it does hurt and I don't like it. I think I'm afraid that if I say anything, fixing the problem will require some kind of procedure and will take a while, and what I want most is to get the hell out of there. Fuck the pain.

And so we are ready to leave (trumpets blare!!). Diana goes to get the car and I am taken down in a wheel-chair. I feel so lousy and so dizzy, that there are moments during the trip down when I want to tell the person pushing me that he had better take me back up, but I don't, and we are outside, Diana is there with the car, and I am on my way home and my cancer is gone. From this moment, as predicted, no more diarrhea, no incontinence, no delusions, no muddy thinking; nothing bad can happen any more. And Diana makes eggs, bacon, potatoes, and toast for lunch. I eat it all, and get into bed.

Soon after, the agency calls to tell us that the nurse assigned to our case quit that morning and they will get someone out to us the next day. They are emphatic; there is no one else available. Diana, the sweet, butter-wouldn't-melt-in her-mouth, catch-a-fly-with-honey, peace advocating, anti-confrontational, saint among mortals, is transformed into Wonder Woman; she is Norma Rae, she is Vivien Leigh swearing that she will never be hungry again, she is Susan Sarandon and Geena Davis blowing away oppressors, and she opens a mouth to the point that you can hear the tremors on the other end. Arrangements are made that a nurse will be over within the hour, and my recuperation begins. No one has taken away her spleen from my beautiful, miraculous wife.

An hour later, Mary comes. I hear her talking to Diana at the entry, she is the early Maureen O'Hara, the lilt of Irish something fills the house and, in my head, strains of *Macushla, Kevin Barry*, and *The Wearing of the Green* accompany her down the corridor as she walks to my bedroom. She's in black, but there is nothing somber about her. She asks how I am feeling; I wax ecstatic. She asks about my nutrition; I tell her what I had for lunch, and she says that that doesn't sound like a sick man. She says that working men eat lunches like that and she questions the necessity of the automatic feeding. But we've been given orders; it seems, as a matter of fact, that it is a condition of the discharge, so she shows Diana how to do it, they set it up and every so often I will be fed automatically. She cleans out my drain; there is almost nothing to clean out, so she wonders why it's still there. She pricks my finger with the little diabetic apparatus I see on TV infomercials, and it's normal. Diana is supposed to do it three times a day, but fortunately we both forget, and since it's always normal when Mary does it, who cares?

I wake up in the morning, with the feeling that something is different. I brush my face with my hand; the feeding tube is gone. Oh shit! It's on my chest. I must have pulled it out during the night. I hated it, I felt it served no function, but I certainly did not intend to pull it out. My unconscious, maybe, but I've been "good" and they can't blame me for what happens in my sleep. You have to prove intention, right? There is no way I can get it back in, I am pleased to say, and when Mary comes she says that there's no point in making a big deal about it; I would have to go back to the hospital and get someone there to insert it and since I'm eating well (and even tasting and enjoying it), who needs the tube. So, no itchy nose, no surrendering control to a tube and timer, no intake of abundant calories without pleasure, and no extra chore for Diana.

Diana calls the food supplement supplier to remove the boxes from our doorway. They did not come when she called before and the boxes are now soaked with rain. This time they say that they will be by the following day and this time they come. But during the night someone has come by and stolen a bunch of the cans. Imagine! Someone coming up ten stairs to steal cans of nutrition supplement from a wet box! But, it's not my problem; I never told them to leave the boxes out of doors and they had been warned.

So now, all Diana's fears are allayed. Everything that has to be done has become almost routine for her and we know now that if we are not sure of anything, Mary will be back and it will get done pleasantly. Mary also mentions that after a week or so she will get a Physical Therapist to come in a few times a week to help me with my wobbliness, my getting up from the couch (a Herculean task for me), my balance, and any other such problems that have come up. Who could ask for anything more, and I am home! My bed, my bathroom, my clothes, my everything, and no one scolds me nor does me anything for my own good. I'm feeling better, gradually spending less time in bed, I'm hungry, and eating well. The physical therapist comes three times a week, devises exercises (that I mostly don't do), works out very practical solutions for activities I'm having trouble with. She pushes me to do more than I want to and, while she's there, at any rate, I do them.

I am to see the surgeon in the midst of all these goodies and he expresses wonderment at how well I look, jokes about my having intended to pull out the tube (I set him straight), seems delighted about everything (I have to admit that I kind of resent his delight; why the hell should I make him happy? I mean, look: my gratitude to this man abounds. He saved my life. He relieved me of a cancer that others had not been able to remove. But I lost a whole bunch of organs, he is patronizing to me, and he intruded himself), and tells me that in a couple of weeks I should have the drain removed. This is indeed a very different visit from the last time I saw him in his office.

After about three weeks, both Mary and the physical therapist decide that I am doing great and don't need their services any longer. I promise each of them that I will continue to practice what they've taught me (my fingers are crossed; I plan nothing of the sort), there are emotional goodbyes (it's amazing how close a sick person comes to be to his care-givers), they are gone and we are on our own I was dying a few weeks ago and now, here we are, taking care of business and ourselves!

The day arrives for the removal of the drain and I am a nervous wreck. A friend, a retired transplant surgery nurse, has explained to me that, because the drain has been in so long, there will be excruciating pain when it is removed.

Paul Singer

She is a very thoughtful, considerate, caring woman, a dear friend, so I figure that there must be some humanitarian concern in her need to tell me this. When she calls me the week of the removal to remind me of how terrible this experience is going to be, I am beginning to question her humanitarian concern, but, by this time, there are an awful lot of people on my shit list, so I try to ignore what she is telling me. Oh sure, just try to ignore it!

My appointment is in Interventional Radiology. I get to the receptionist, who very apologetically, very warmly, with a beautiful Russian accent, with empathy for my plight tells me that according to their records (and a phone call she just made) the appointment is for the other Interventional Radiology halfway across the city and that there is no way I can make it in time; but because my papers give this address, (and because she is straight out of Chekhov) she will see whether it is possible, given their very busy schedule, to have it done right there. I wait maybe ten minutes, a woman comes out, and, with considerable grace, escorts me to the area, where three women, with enormous charm and humor, fawn over me and set me up for the procedure. The radiologist herself enters, I tell her about the warning about pain that I've been given and the expectation that I have, she reassures me that I need not be concerned, it's not their experience that patients suffer much pain. They inject a local anesthetic in my side; because the injection itself hurts more that I expect, I tighten up with tension to the point that I think I'm three or four inches above the table, and the radiologist tells me that the tube is out. I didn't feel the removal! After these women reject my proposal of marriage, the radiologist tells me that the tube was rubbing against my rib and that that was the source of the pain that I was feeling in certain positions. When the nurse had jerked the tube, it changed its position. So there we are. No more pain, no need for alertness about how I position myself.

And now, for the moment anyway, free at last.

XII

*In which I reflect on some of my experiences when
unclothed before new doctors and find myself
grateful for my survival, whatever it took*

Now a couple of small observations or reflections that I've saved for last and then I'll wrap this up.

Even prior to the most recent surgery, I had, as you certainly will remember, something of (at least to me) an impressive abdominal scar. You would also very likely agree that my current lack of a left kidney is an item that is surely one of the highlights of my medical career and hence my medical records. I mean, it's not every day that you meet somebody, one of whose kidneys has been removed. It has, I would think, some considerable dramatic punch. Why is it then that every time I see a new doctor, to whom my medical records are certainly available and on whom I haven't suddenly nor by chance stumbled, (that is, he/she certainly has had a moment or two to review my file, however cursorily—my being there is invariably a scheduled appointment!), when that doctor has access to my belly, he/she invariably says to me something like, "What's that scar? Did you have your gall bladder removed?" I always am a little embarrassed for them when I say, "No, I had a radical nephrectomy," and then they say, "Oh, of course," like they knew it all the time.

This is not only a frequent happening; there has been no exception! Could it be that they refrain from looking at records because they like to meet the patient fresh, with no prior knowledge, as though real information might bias their diagnostic judgment? Or are they simply too rushed to go over even the highlights of a patient's record? Or is it simply carefree abandon? Whatever the reason, this does not deliver much confidence to the scar owner.

Here's the other one. I have a brightly colored tattoo of a coiled snake on my right hip, toward the back. When my pants are down just a few inches and you approach me from the right or from the back, it is very difficult to miss it. No, it is impossible to miss it. While tattoos these days are commonplace, they are rare in people like me.There is no doubt that I am a nice, educated, elderly, Jewish professional man, born in the thirties, came of age in the fifties, I am politically liberal, opposed to war, and interested in "the finer things"—I read Jane Austen and Philip Roth, I love Fra Angelico, Piero della Francesca, and I even know a lot about Frank Stella, I do not own a baseball cap, I have not been to prison; none of these easily observable attributes of mine jibes quite with my having a coiled snake on my hip. One might think, therefore, that there would be at least a touch of curiosity in the viewer when the tattoo is exposed. So why has nobody, not one person, within the medical establishment, many of whom have had ample view of my right hip toward the back, ever commented or asked me about the tattoo? Not one! Never! (Well, actually one person I mentioned a while back, a lower level nursing assistant, did comment on it—but only one). Could they think that the question might be somewhat too personal, even though they are examining or doing things to areas of my body that I would certainly see as personal? They think

Paul Singer

nothing, for example, of pressing their hands into what I see as private areas of my body, but curiosity about an artifact on my skin is taboo?

I would certainly wonder what the story is if I saw someone like me with a tattoo like mine and, if I felt comfortable enough, I would ask about it. But then, maybe that's the thing, that they don't feel comfortable connecting with me about an attribute of mine that, however blatant it may be, is not essentially medical in nature. Could I say that this might reflect a reluctance to engage on a personal, human level? What I find surprising, given the number of medical personnel who have had access to my backside, is the absolute consistency with which questions about the tattoo are avoided.

There may be, though, another side to this coin. Perhaps there are two kinds of tattooed people in the world: those who don't mind their tattoos commented on in a medical setting and those who do, and how is the practitioner to know in advance whose hip he's looking at. Maybe no comment is the easiest, least offensive way out of the dilemma. Maybe, maybe not.

Almost every time that I tell anybody any of the anecdotes that I've narrated here, the response has been, "You think that's strange? Listen to what happened to me (or to a friend of mine or to an aunt)." This too is an absolutely uniform and consistent response. It seems that everybody has had or knows somebody who has had strange and disappointing encounters with the medical system. I am not talking here about the sub-standard, third world medical care that we unfortunately expect for people living in poverty. I am talking about technically first-rate medicine (securely paid for, of course, by insurance) delivered in uncaring, dehumanized, impersonal, thoughtless ways.

Apparently the learning that first year medical students did in that course I mentioned at the beginning of my story about how to talk and listen to patients (that is, how to empathize with them), that I was part of way back then, was forgotten in their clinical years in medical school and in residencies! People learn to think and operate the way their mentors do and this unfortunately is the result; professional attitudes perpetuate themselves. That's just the way that professions work! Apprentices learn from their superiors. No doubt about any of that, but I for one have trouble adapting to it. Maybe we're talking here about my rigidity (you've got to learn to swing with the punches, they say), my need to have things just the way I would design them. I don't know.

People have told me that I react to medical issues in the same way that I react to everything else around me—and I agree: I'm impatient, I'm critical, I give equal weight to small inconveniences and important events, I notice everything and read too much into things going on around me, I try to understand the meaning of my interactions, I am quick to anger. I have, as you have surely noticed (and, I hope, forgiven) a penchant for expletives and gutter words; that is simply how I think and talk (might as well be how I write). All that is true. Clearly I am the same person in every situation I encounter. I am not easy. I expect a lot. I enter these medical encounters anticipating that the personnel is eager to know me and help me. I am an optimistic fellow and when events don't meet my expectations I am disappointed and then tend to be critical. But, I am not fabricating the events themselves and the inconveniences that I describe. And it certainly makes sense to me to feel that in areas as important as one's health, one's very life and, perhaps, death, even nuisances gain importance. In the medical arena, as in most human interactions, there is a lot of meaning in nuance. The devil, for me, has always been in the details.

My view here is that minor inconveniences mirror an attitude that creates larger problems. If the institution expends little energy in making the visit convenient and comfortable (eg. doesn't use signage that truly enables one to find one's way, doesn't have a no waiting policy, doesn't train staff to recognize that patients are people with feelings, etc.), it is an institution that is not respectful of its clients; and if *it* is not respectful of its clients, those who work for that institution will not be respectful of their clients, and from there, the disrespect spirals. It should be clear then that when one is being cared for, the trappings of caring should be evident. As far as I am concerned, *care* mandates that feelings, meanings on a personal level, the whole business of dignity for the patient ought to be on everyone's mind. All personnel ought to be cognizant of the fact that every interaction with a patient is a transaction between two people.

It is well to keep in mind that these events, these conditions that I talk about (and that scores of people tell me about) did not occur in only one medical institution; nor did they happen in just one state. They happened (and happen) all over the place: teaching hospitals, managed care facilities, private, independent practitioners, just about any kind of urban setting where medical things take place. It is certainly not one institution, not one kind of institution, nor one geographic locale that is the locus of these problems. I know that it is not just my luck. These problems are surely endemic in the delivery of medical care in this country.

Maybe medical practitioners (not just doctors: I am talking about nurses, technicians of all kinds, anybody who deals with sick people in a "helping" capacity, that is, people in what is frequently, perhaps ingenuously, perhaps humorously, called the *caring* professions) ought to learn a thing or two about empathy and reciprocity or at the very least to think about the meaning to the patient of what they are about to do or say, before it is done or said. Here's an example of a problem communication: about two weeks before she died, I'm standing by Sandra's bed in the ICU, she is, as she has been for a while now, minimally responsive, I stay fifteen minutes or so, pretending to have a conversation with her, I get up to leave and one of the nurses I barely know indicates that she wants to speak to me; I approach her and she says, "Mr. Singer, don't you think you're being a little selfish keeping her alive like this, on a respirator?" Hard to believe, this introduction, isn't it, but that is how it happened.

We all know, or at least have read, that the death of a spouse is extremely stressful; it's a huge loss and somehow the surviving spouse, at some point along the way, has to accept it, allow it. So, this nurse is surely right and this is a conversation that certainly should be taking place, but it's not going to, I'm afraid, when the intro is an accusation that I cannot help but interpret as an attack and to which I am sure to react defensively.

Nobody has brought this subject up to me before and, foolish or not, I have not let myself begin to think about—from my point of view, at that moment—sanctioning her death, causing her death, killing her (my beautiful, beloved, forty-five year old wife of twenty-five years, married to me more than half her young life, is dying and I can't stand that; now, out of the blue, I'm supposed to feel guilty that I don't pull her plug?). I don't realize that there is not a specific event or moment that is supposed to initiate

257

that line of thinking and I view the nurse's statement as a put-down, rather than as an opening for an important discussion because in fact it is a put-down.

I respond with some ridiculous defensive statement (prior to my escaping to the stairwell to sob) and nothing comes out of this very brief interaction, except that I feel terrible about myself, about my selfishness causing Sandra these most undignified few weeks and allowing the situation to continue another two weeks, and the nurse very likely feels either that she's flubbed an important transaction or that I am a monstrous fool. Nothing constructive happens! The conversation that should take place never occurs.

What I expect from medical people may be a little subtle. It's not friendship I want of these people, my doctors. I don't need them to share my taste in movies and music. I don't even need them to be of the same political or philosophical point of view. What I need is, that, while they are in there with me, they be genuine, that they be interested in me, that they care about me, that there be some ability and wish to empathize with me, to put themselves, at least for the moments that we are together, in my shoes, that they communicate openly and honestly with me about what their thinking is about my situation and that the communication be specifically to me, in their own way, not from a script, that they care whether I live or die, and that, when I die, there even be a tear or two. I would even like them to grapple with whether or not to attend my funeral. It's by no means important that they attend; it's the grappling I want. From my own clinical work I know how great the burden is on the clinician when these expectations are met, how costly it is emotionally, how much work is required. But if it's not there, the patients, the consumers, are woefully out of luck; they are short-changed.

Now here's another thing that doctors do that I think has ramifications. Some time ago, I noticed that when a physician friend of mine referred to any patients he was treating he would say "a person I take care of" ("What is he talking about," I thought. "He's an ophthalmologist. He's dealing only with eyes") and then I began to notice that phrase when other physicians in my circle talked about patients. Being a psychologist, I have to insist that what people say reflects something about how they see things. I don't think it can be tossed off merely as a semantic issue and that they don't really mean something by it. For me, words do have meaning and these doctors are saying that those people whose illnesses or medical problems they treat are theirs to be cared for.

I find this a strange concept indeed. I would never say, for example, that teachers take care of children in their classroom; nannies, maybe, but only during the absence of their parents. *Taking care* of (not *giving care* to) someone means assuming authority over that person who, for whatever reason, cannot exercise responsibility on his/her own. A normal adult person *takes care* of him/herself; he/she asks a doctor to figure out and/or treat a particular problem that has developed, but does not surrender responsibility or competence to anybody. One doesn't usually feel that a professional whom you consult is taking care of you; maybe *taking care* of a problem of yours, but not of you. But even that!

It seems to me that the phrase has to define something about the way the doctor sees his relationship to the patient whose problem he is diagnosing or treating. There is at least a concept of authority to which the patient is supposed to acquiesce. This authority is by no means malicious; it may even be loving. But it is certainly not the service (or attitude) that I am asking for, nor is it what my insurance pays for. So long as I am sentient, aware, competent, nobody takes care of me, except myself and, on occasion, when I want it, my wife. There are subtle issues of control here and I think that what is being communicated is a message to the patient that demands some kind of passivity.

A doctor with the greatest technical proficiency who cannot empathize or isn't willing to empathize might do better to stay in a lab somewhere and not minister to people, because if there is no emotional reciprocity, he may be doing them harm. After all these medical contacts of mine, after all the doctoring, after all this time, I know from my experience that being seen as an organ system, as something other than a person, can be destructive, it can hurt the spirit. And that is particularly damaging from those people who we expect will be helpful to us. I know things are going well between us, that it is a trusting relationship, when I notice, for example, that Charlie is a little disappointed that I am not as observant a Jew as he would like me to be; he knows who I am, he lets me know who he is—we are two people in a humanly meaningful interaction. That defines, for me, the context in which the best medical care for me can take place.

I feel a little foolish, a little awkward being critical of medical systems that I have encountered as a patient, because when you really get down to it, here's the thing: my eyes may be puffy, I may have been injecting myself weekly with Procrit, I may be napping every day, but I am alive, I feel good, and I am functioning well. I am never out of breath, and I can walk as far as I want to (uphill will always be a problem—it always has been!). During a four and a half year period, when getting up, I had to sit on the edge of the bed for a while before standing to avoid feeling woozy, out of breath, bad; during those four and a half years, when I stood up at the end of a movie, I had to brace myself against a side wall until those sensations went away; for four and a half years I had to make plans in everything that I did—everything!—to avoid or at least lessen those frightening feelings. And now I skip through everything without needing to think. These changes are very big numbers for me—and I know that I did not get to this place by myself. I am aware and grateful every hour of every day for doctors who worked with me, for modern medicine, combined perhaps with my own unrelenting commitment to participate in and understand any decisions being made about me.

I feel strongly, in retrospect, that I could have avoided some of the problems in my story. I should, for example, have put off my kidney surgery a few weeks and gone in to talk with the surgeon once more in order to get more specific information about his plans for the procedure. If all the signs looked so bad to me, and the surgery itself had to be squeezed into his schedule, it was foolish on my part to go blithely ahead with it. I should probably have stopped Interferon long before I did; it was doing me no good and the side-effects were dreadful. Those, for starters. But it's hard to make rational decisions under this kind of stress—you feel that if you don't do it immediately and if you don't keep at it—as though just one more dose will be the one that is going to fix you up—you're going to die. So I can't fault myself too much.

I am, though, very proud of my resolution to rid myself of my medical problems—I never thought of myself as a cancer patient, a cancer victim, or a cancer survivor; my view always is that I am a man with certain diseases that I have to do something about. I could never, for example, be in a cancer support group, because there, the identification of me as a sufferer of the disease is prominent and essential and I can't think of myself that way. (This is not, by the way, a quality that I always admire about myself. I know that it is defensive and may even be magical, as though if we don't mention its name, I'm essentially free of it. And also, the attitude leads to resentment and tension in me whenever any well-intending person, who knows my recent history, asks me how I am feeling. They ask graciously, and I interpret condescension and pity; I often even begin to respond with displeasure, but mostly I am able to catch myself. This wife of mine is an angel to put up with some of my shtick! Hooray for love!)

It seems to me from this vantage point that very likely most of the medical practitioners I have had contact with—certainly and unfortunately, however, not all of them—did their best medically or pretty close to their best with me; but it is absolutely clear to me that that is very far from enough. Civility, humanity, an awareness of who I am and how I feel, making my trip through the system easy and rational, are prerequisites, they are the bases on which medical care should be delivered, and a significant number of doctors I dealt with had it in spades. Otherwise, and too often, I am a piece of meat.

I started to write about these events as a way to put my experience into perspective, for me and for anyone who might be interested. In most respects nowadays, I am a very happy man, I am unencumbered, I am free, I am in charge of my experience and in ways that count, as much as is possible, in control of my medical care. I plan to keep myself in that position as long as I am able to and one thing I've learned from all this is that I will not return for a second visit ever again to physicians or others in the medical system who do not enable me to continue to feel that way. None of us should.

So let me end with a little advice. Any time you get sick, make sure that you understand what is happening, not only in your body (don't stop asking questions until you are sure that you understand, take notes, write it down), but also with the medical people who are involved—that is, what they are thinking and where that thinking leads, and, please, be prepared to acknowledge your fears, even at the first symptoms, and stay vigilant about what is going on. Use the Internet and libraries. Talk to people, read books, use the internet. Be in as much control as you can be, try to surrender as little control as you are able to. Ask questions, solicit answers that clarify issues for you, above all, make sure to put yourself in a position that enables you to make choices. When possible, if you are to be hospitalized, try to arrange that it be scheduled so that your stay not include a weekend and that it be long before or after important holidays: hospitals are understaffed at those times and you want all the staff they can afford. Keep in mind too that July is when new residents start; by winter they are likely to be doing their thing better. Use the knowledge your doctors have, listen to the advice they give and their rational explanations, but *you* make the choices. At least, that's a beginning—a significant move toward getting humane care.

Please, above all, take care of yourself and be well. I wish you good health.

L'chaim!